Counselling skills
IN PALLIATIVE CARE

John Davy and Susan Ellis

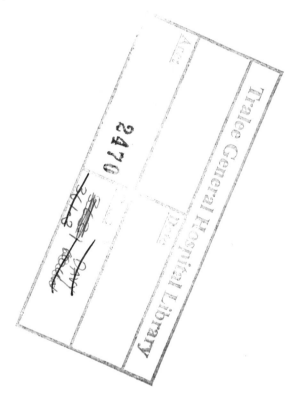

Open University Press
Buckingham · Philadelphia

Open University Press
Celtic Court
22 Ballmoor
Buckingham
MK18 1XW

email: enquiries@openup.co.uk
world wide web: www.openup.co.uk

and
325 Chestnut Street
Philadelphia, PA 19106, USA

First Published 2000
Reprinted 2002

ISBN   0 335 20312 4 (pb)   0 335 20313 2 (hb)

A catalogue record of this book is available from the British Library

Library of Congress Cataloging-in-Publication Data
Davy, John, 1965–
        Counselling skills in palliative care / by John Davy and Susan Ellis.
        p. cm.
        Includes bibliographical references and index.
        ISBN 0-335-20312-4 (pb) – ISBN 0-335-20313-2 (hb)
        1. Palliative treatment. 2. Terminally ill–Counseling of. 3. Terminal
care. I. Ellis, Susan, 1966– II. Title.
        R726.8.D29 2000
        616 .029–dc21
                                                                                00-035626

Copy-edited and typeset by The Running Head Limited,
www.therunninghead.com
Printed in Great Britain by The Cromwell Press, Trowbridge

€23·40

Counselling skills
IN PALLIATIVE CARE

Our thanks to Rob, Ruth and Jane

Contents

Chapter **1**   Introduction   1

Chapter **2**   Joining the palliative care system   17

Chapter **3**   Empowering patients, finding goals and
                   resources   31

Chapter **4**   Living with loss   49

Chapter **5**   Symptom management   69

Chapter **6**   Anger   83

Chapter **7**   Palliative care and children   99

Chapter **8**   Dying and death itself   111

Chapter **9**   Bereavement support   123

Chapter **10**   Caring: the privilege and the price   134

Chapter **11**   Developing counselling skills   148

Chapter **12**   Concluding remarks   158

Appendix A: Using family genograms   161
Appendix B: Contacts and resources   169
References   177
Index   182

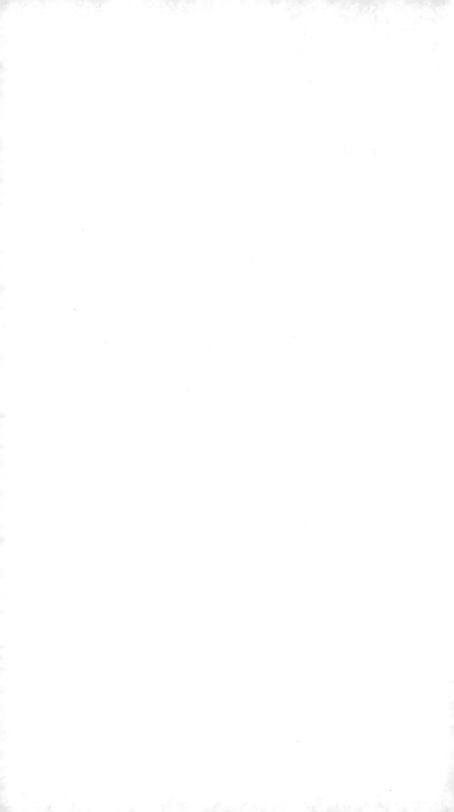

Chapter 1

Introduction

Case note 1

Linda walked unsteadily out of the hospital doors, wandering over to the car park as if in a dream. She sat in the car for almost an hour without turning the engine on, tears streaming down her face and breathing raggedly. She kept hearing the doctor's words again and again: 'I am very sorry, Miss Henry, I really am. I'm afraid there is nothing more that we can do.' 'What am I going to do?' she asked herself over and over. 'What am I going to tell the children? Why me, why terminal cancer? Shit, shit, shit.'

This is a book about counselling skills that healthcare professionals (HCPs) can use in their work in palliative care. We begin our book by outlining the development of palliative care within the UK since the modern hospice movement began, and comment on the different and sometimes problematic meanings of terms such as 'hospice care' and 'palliative care'. We introduce the reader to some of the complexities facing HCPs working in teams to provide palliative care, and to the major existential dilemmas which are likely to face people dealing with life-threatening illness. The last part of the chapter offers a conceptual framework for thinking about counselling skills and supportive roles in palliative care which we will draw on in the rest of the book. Subsequent chapters use clinical examples drawn from different stages of palliative care to explore these issues, and offer practical guidance on the use of counselling skills to enhance the supportive roles of professional helpers in palliative care.

What is palliative care?

There has been a rapid development of medical science and technology over the last century, leading to the virtual eradication of many lethal or disabling conditions in the Western world. Each year seems to bring news of another discovery, drug or treatment with which to challenge illness and disease. There have been substantial gains in the average expected lifespan for citizens fortunate enough to live in countries sufficiently wealthy to benefit from medical advances, improved nutrition and better public hygiene.

However, death still comes to us all. Twentieth-century biomedical science was particularly successful against acute conditions and infectious diseases, thanks largely to the discovery of antibiotic agents. Instead, we are increasingly likely to die from chronic and progressive illnesses such as the cancers, coronary and circulatory diseases, dementias and other degenerative conditions. At the same time, improvements in diagnostic accuracy have outpaced the development of curative treatments, so that patients and families may now face an extended period of living with the knowledge that the patient has an incurable and progressive condition.

Sometimes medical advances may actually worsen the position of those with incurable conditions. For instance, there may be tantalizing glimpses of possible cures under investigation, but too new to help today's patients. Effective treatments may be known but unavailable because of cost or other considerations. Modern multidrug treatments for HIV/AIDS are increasingly effective, but too expensive for many in less developed nations, or counterindicated for patients with advanced disease who have already been exposed to less sophisticated drug therapy regimes. Their long-term utility remains uncertain.

Doctors and others in the helping and caring professions

face a twin challenge in supporting those affected by progressive and potentially fatal diseases such as cancer, motor neurone disease (MND) and AIDS. First, what else can be done to eliminate or to prevent conditions which are currently untreatable – in other words, to extend the patient's life in purely quantitative terms? Second, what can be done to improve the quality of remaining life and the manner of dying for those who cannot be cured, together with supporting their family and friends? This latter question is the central concern of palliative care.

It is sometimes difficult and can be downright unwise to make a clear distinction between palliative care and treatment which still aims at cure, particularly since it is not possible to predict the future course of many diseases with certainty. A patient with a diagnosis of lung cancer may still hope that their treatment will cure them, even if they appreciate that the odds are against their long-term survival. Such a patient may benefit from concurrent treatments aimed at both their overall quantity and quality of life. The treatment emphasis would shift in response to changes in the disease process, whether this be towards a lengthy or indefinite remission, or towards a terminal phase. The difference between palliative care and other interventions is perhaps best understood as one of emphasis and priorities, rather than an absolute distinction.

These ambiguities can be confusing. Newcomers to palliative care – including of course most patients and families – may be unsure about the different terms used by professionals such as 'palliative care', 'hospice care' and 'terminal care'. Even among experienced workers in the field, there may be disagreements. Some of these differences reflect historical patterns in the development of the field, and the philosophical stances and value positions taken by different workers (NCHSPCS 1995).

The development of palliative care

'Hospice care' draws on a long tradition of caring, harking back to the hospitallers of medieval Europe who offered care and rest – hospitality – to pilgrims passing through. The early pioneers of palliative care in Britain such as Cicely Saunders chose this term carefully. They wanted to emphasize a relationship in which care, not simply medical treatment, is freely given without attempting to change the traveller's eventual destination. The aim is to respect and support the patient's journey, not for the patient to meet the institution's goals. There is also an implicit suggestion in the term that we travel through life, and perhaps beyond death, with purpose and meaning. This need not be framed in conventional religious terms, but certainly represents an emphasis on the care of the soul as well as the body.

The modern hospice movement in Britain was initially developed outside the NHS in the 1960s by Saunders and others, who believed that existing NHS facilities were overly concerned with an attempt to arrest or cure disease processes through medical treatments, viewing death mainly in negative terms as a failure of treatment. Cicely Saunders wrote her first paper on caring for the dying person in 1957, and the first hospice, St Christopher's in London, opened a decade later. Hospices occupied buildings separate from hospitals and cancer wards, with their own staff comprising teams of nurses, therapists, chaplains, social workers and doctors. As a part of the deliberate 'demedicalization' or 'deprofessionalization' of dying and death, the early hospices welcomed a substantial involvement of volunteers from the local community. Of course, the struggle to ensure adequate funding for the early hospices may also have been a factor in the decision to use this unpaid support.

This care was established mainly for cancer patients with a short life expectancy, with the aim of attending to the patient as a person rather than a problem. Death was seen as an event or process which could be supported and even valued, not as a foe to be resisted at all costs. Medical treatments had a place in relieving and managing distressing symptoms, but as part of a broader approach to care. Hospices emphasized the importance of creating a safe and supportive environment, creating opportunities for talking, listening and reflection, and helping patients to remain as independent and creative as possible. Hospices also aimed to work with the family of the patient who were seen both as a valuable part of the caring team and as people who might themselves be in need of support both before and after the patient's death.

The original independent hospices established sufficient credibility that several NHS hospices were later founded to emulate their apparent success in addressing quality of life issues for those with progressive, eventually fatal, diseases. Although most hospices were primarily established for patients with advanced cancer, they have also developed a role in supporting patients with other progressive and incurable diseases such as motor neurone disease and multiple sclerosis (Tebbitt 1999). With the advent of AIDS in the 1980s, some hospices began offering beds to those suffering from this new disease, and some specialist AIDS hospice facilities were founded.

Although the early hospice movement established a formidable reputation, several limitations became apparent. For example, they were unable to offer support to more than a tiny percentage of patients with advanced incurable disease in the UK. In effect they helped raise some of the standards expected in the field and redefined the range of care needed by patients and families, but without then being able to meet the needs of the wider population thus identified. Furthermore, the initial development of hospice care within specialist organizations set apart from mainstream healthcare may sometimes have encouraged a belief that hospice care is not so much a philosophy relevant to any health setting, but instead is a minority interest pursued only by specialists in hospice buildings.

Combined with a perception that many patients would like to be supported in their own homes rather than an institutional setting, a drive developed to extend services and care to patients staying mainly at home, and to patients still receiving treatment through hospital departments (Tebbitt 1999). Hospices have increasingly provided day-care services and out-patient facilities, and sought a role as trainers and consultants to other professionals involved in providing palliative care to patients, such as GPs, district nurses and hospital departments.

The early hospices emphasized their role in supporting patients who were dying. However, as medical treatments for the underlying conditions developed (e.g. more effective chemotherapy for cancer patients, and multidrug treatments for AIDS patients), it became increasingly apparent that many patients with progressive and incurable disease might live for years rather than weeks or months. In-patient beds for the imminently dying in hospices (those in a 'terminal phase' of illness) did not adequately address these needs, leading to more emphasis on supporting people to 'live with' their disease, rather than 'die well' despite the disease.

The term 'palliative care' has evolved to reflect these shifts towards supporting patients and families in a broader range of settings than the traditional in-patient hospice. Although the need to provide terminal care remains an important part of palliative care, there is perhaps a greater emphasis on the relief of symptoms and improvement of quality of life.

The 1985 decision of the Royal College of Physicians to recognize a new medical specialism of 'Palliative Care Consultant' can be seen partly as a recognition by the medical profession of the lessons the hospice movement had to teach, but also partly as an attempt by the medical establishment to reclaim this field for medical treatment rather than holistic care. This distinction is sometimes captured in choices to rename NHS 'palliative care' units as 'palliative medicine' departments.

Some long-time supporters of the hospice ethos have expressed concern that 'palliative care' may be a slippery slope leading back to the remedicalization of the care of dying patients, with a renewed focus on increasingly active and technical measures to provide symptom relief at the expense of a more holistic emphasis on the human experience of patient and family, and arguably less emphasis on death itself. Biswas (1993) argues that there is a danger that death itself could be treated simply as another inconvenient symptom which could one day be 'palliated' or somehow made 'painless'.

Of course, the public perception of hospices and palliative care is affected by these historical trends. Some patients who might benefit from careful attention to symptom control, perhaps still with a prognosis of months or even years, may be very reluctant to enter a hospice even for a short admission, fearing instead that 'that's the place where you go to die – you come out of there feet first'.

Case note 2

Alice was a 35-year-old woman experiencing considerable pain from bony metastases secondary to breast cancer. Her mother, May, had died from breast cancer some 25 years previously, after a difficult period of distressing constipation, nausea and stupor shortly after she began taking morphine. The GP had a good relationship with Alice and managed to persuade Alice that commencing morphine did not mean 'the end of the road'. Unfortunately, Alice herself reacted very poorly to MST tablets (morphine), becoming confused and nauseous. The GP wanted Alice to go to the local hospice for a short admission to review pain medication options, but Alice refused point-blank, saying only: 'I'm not ready to die yet, they'll just put me down like a dog in there.'

Conversely, the developing emphasis on 'symptom relief' in palliative care may inadvertently encourage a resurgence of unhelpful euphemism between patients, family and professionals when death is very near, but open discussion of this is avoided.

Case note 3

Fred was a farmer in his seventies with a tumour in his throat that was progressively obstructing his airways and also making it painful for him to eat and drink. He had been admitted to hospital as an emergency following an episode of choking which frightened and distressed Fred and his wife Fran very badly. Fred's medication was changed in the hospital which seemed to help relieve his breathing difficulties, but it was clear that he was becoming increasingly tired and experiencing greater pain on swallowing. Fred's adult children Harris and Gill could see that he was becoming very gaunt and changing colour and wondered if he was about to die, but could not find a way to share their thoughts with either of their parents, who accepted the hospital consultant's suggestion that Fred 'go down to the hospice for a week or two to help you both get some energy back, and get that pain under control so you can eat again'.

Such apparent avoidance would directly oppose the hospice founders' vision that only by directly confronting death as a taboo could the fear of it be relieved and the needs of the dying directly addressed. Although modern palliative care aims towards effective symptom control and improving quality of life, this must complement rather than replace the goal of supporting death as a natural and dignified human process. Professionals supporting patients and families in palliative care need to consider carefully not just what their own understanding and intentions are in palliative care, but also how this fits with the expectations and beliefs of those they care for.

The complexity of multidisciplinary team work

Modern palliative care services, whether delivered through hospice units or community-based teams, use the capabilities of many different professionals. These might include nurses, doctors, counsellors and complementary therapists, psychologists, occupational and physiotherapists, clergy, managers, volunteers, administration staff and social workers. Behind the scenes, many other staff such as cleaners and pharmacists provide vital support to the palliative care approach. In larger hospices, these professionals may be a part of a multidisciplinary team which meets regularly. In smaller units or in community teams there may be a core of key workers, such as the GP and their practice staff together with the district nursing team, supported by input from other professionals as requested (and of course as available, area to area).

To be able to help effectively, there must be good communication and working alliances between these many different professionals, the patient and their family/carers, and possibly also the hospital team if a patient still needs oncology-based services, palliative surgical measures or specialist pain clinic intervention. Although on the one hand patients and their families may welcome the idea that there are many different professionals who may be able to offer support, there are also risks that care may be fragmented or overly intrusive, precisely because so many different people may be involved. The following are some of the more common problems that may arise.

- Existing good relations between patient/family and GP may be disrupted because of the intervention of so many others.
- The life of the patient/family may be disrupted because of too many appointments and consultations with different professionals, with little time and energy left for anything else.
- There may be mixed, unclear or conflicting messages from different professionals to the patient/family, or within the professional team. Patients and families may sometimes find themselves struggling to interpret and translate between the differing professional 'languages' spoken by clergy, nurses, doctors and counsellors, even when these professionals feel that they are working well together.
- Each professional may be looking after 'their bit' of the patient/family's care, without anyone establishing a relationship with the patient/family as whole people rather than problems to be treated. This may be particularly damaging since the patient and family may already feel that they are being 'pulled to pieces' by the disease itself, by medical interventions, and by the stress of living with illness.
- The needs of some patients or family/carers may slip through the gaps in the net of care as each professional assumes that someone else is 'dealing with that bit' (Davy 1999). This can be a particular risk for family members and other carers, as many professionals are trained, at least initially, to focus their support on the patient who is identified as having the problem – the disease itself. Even where professionals aim to 'involve' the family, this can sometimes mean using the family as a resource to support the professional's own planned intervention with the patient, rather than to support the family. Further problems may arise if the professional team's definition of a 'family' differs substantially from the patient's, for example through cross-cultural misunderstandings (Carter and McGoldrick 1999).
- Members of the professional team may find it hard to gauge the value of their work and gain job satisfaction which can sustain them, if they do not have an ongoing relationship with the patient or the family beyond their own period of 'intervention'. Without such feedback, professionals may experience disillusionment or burn-out, or inadvertently continue unhelpful practices.

The dilemmas faced by patients and families in palliative care

---

Case note 4

A few months later, Linda asked the nurse at her GP practice: 'Do you think I should ask to go on this experimental course of chemotherapy the oncologist mentioned? I feel very tired and I'm frightened it'll be even worse than the other course I had, but I don't want to let my children down, I've got to take every chance, haven't I?' She started crying again, and shook with fear.

Case note 5

Thelma had been a professional singer all her adult life. Treatment for a cancer of the larynx led to a tracheotomy and the loss of her beautiful singing voice. Palliative radiotherapy treatment relieved her pain from bony metastases well, but she took to her bed and seemed very depressed, writing in an elegant copperplate for a district nurse that: 'I wish you people had just cut my head right off and got it over with quickly. I've got nothing left.' Her partner Cassie grew increasingly anxious and angry: 'She's just wasting the time we've got left together. I can't make her see that I still love her and need her. I don't want her to give up, but it breaks my heart to see her just lying there.'

The range of difficulties that may be faced by patients and families over the course of a progressive illness such as incurable cancer are extensive but also highly variable. Important factors will include the type and stage of the disease, existing patterns of relationships and resources in the family, the life-cycle stage of the individual and family, and the information and treatments that are potentially available in the local community, including of course the particular personalities, 'style' and skills of HCPs who may become involved. These themes will be explored further through the examples in the rest of the book.

However, it is possible to identify four major dilemmas or anxieties which are likely to be present in some form for all those caught up in the drama and tragedy of a life-threatening illness. These are, in a sense, common human 'existential' dilemmas which potentially face us all throughout life, but which we tend to push to the back of our mind when we are well and happy. The psychotherapist Irving Yalom has written an excellent collection of short stories (Yalom 1989) which illustrates these existential themes very movingly. Illness and uncertainty tend to bring these issues powerfully to the fore.

- Isolation: patients and carers can feel extremely isolated, lonely and vulnerable. There may be a literal isolation, as illness prevents contact with former colleagues and friends, or death takes away a partner, or the progressive isolation of 'alienation' as the experience of the patient becomes increasingly bound up with themes of illness and treatment, and more 'remote' from that of healthy friends and relatives.
- Meaninglessness: patients and carers may find it hard to see what meaning or purpose is left in their life if they believe they will die soon. This feeling may be particularly acute if the physical consequences of illness have severely restricted the options and activities once most important to the patient. Thelma's inability to sing was causing deep distress to her and her partner.
- Choice: it may seem odd to claim that 'choice' can be a dilemma or a cause of distress, especially since HCPs are usually trained to try to maximize patients' sense of autonomy and independence. However, choices in the context of a life-threatening illness may have particular difficult qualities. With time 'running out', choosing one action or person may effectively mean rejecting another, without an opportunity to make amends or correct mistakes later. Many 'choices' in this context may be very emotionally charged, have long-lasting consequences, and require decisions in the face of massive uncertainty. Linda's agonized question reflects this dilemma.

- Death: many aspects of good palliative care are akin to the sensitive and caring support necessary for rehabilitation and long-term disability, but palliative care also implies an acceptance, at least by the professional team, that death is a part of the journey. How can we imagine, prepare or 'come to terms' with this unique event?

These existential anxieties may be expressed and experienced in different ways and to different degrees at particular times for any given patient and family. Fear, anxiety, anger, guilt and sadness may all be present, although sometimes in relatively 'disguised' or unacknowledged ways.

Counselling skills in palliative care

We hope that this book will help to illustrate how good use of counselling skills by HCPs is an important part of supporting patients, relatives and carers through the journey of a life-threatening and progressive illness. We believe that an essential foundation to this work is a recognition of our common humanity, and an awareness that much of what we can offer is through our relationship with others, not simply what we can do to others. This requires us not just to be professionals, but also to be persons. As such, we have our own vulnerabilities, weaknesses and needs for support, and a capacity to receive as well as offer help. After all, we are all on the same journey towards death, simply at different points on the path and with different baggage. Consequently, we hope that this book will also suggest how counselling skills can help professionals work with and support each other, and perhaps also highlight how we can allow patients and those close to them to help us.

What do we mean by 'counselling skills'?

There are of course many different approaches to counselling and therapy, such as the person-centred, psychodynamic, cognitive, existential and systemic models. Each of these orientations to therapeutic work has its own preferred ways of working, its own specific skills. We do not assume that readers would want to become counsellors or psychotherapists, and this book is not designed to teach a specific counselling model. (For readers who wish to begin a more detailed study of particular models of therapy, Woolfe and Dryden (1996) provides a concise but sophisticated discussion of different approaches.) However, there is a growing body of research on counselling which points towards the value of certain common factors and skills which seem to underpin all effective therapeutic work across the different counselling models (Miller *et al.* 1997). In particular, it seems crucial that helpers should:

- clarify and work with the client's goals;
- emphasize the resources and competencies of clients, not simply their difficulties;
- pay attention to the context of the problems and the possible solutions, recognizing that factors and events outside the therapeutic relationship itself may have a very significant impact on the possibilities for change (e.g. changes in the physical disease process, changes within the family network such as a new grandchild);
- offer support through a relationship (Rogers 1957) which the client experiences as:
  - non-judgemental
  - genuine, without the helpers pretending or deceiving the client or themselves, and which respects and values them unconditionally as a whole person (without necessarily supporting or agreeing with all their views or behaviour). This 'respect' is termed 'unconditional positive regard' in some approaches to therapy (such as person-centred counselling) to distinguish it from conditional valuing of the form: 'I will respect you if you do/are xyz . . .'
- help the client to make sense of their current experiences in relation to their core beliefs and values; and
- help the client to develop and sustain some kind of hope for the future.

We regard these as the core counselling skills which HCPs should offer to patients and families as a part of holistic palliative care. It is important to keep these clearly in mind when considering how to use particular techniques such as active listening, questioning, giving feedback, reframing, and so on. In the chapters that follow, we provide a series of clinical vignettes to illustrate how these high-level skills may be implemented in specific cases, and to suggest how palliative care workers can try to manage the dilemmas and difficulties that may arise.

Counselling skills can be seen as the intentional use of a relationship to provide support to a person in distress. This may or may not be concurrent with the use of other supportive procedures such as medication, massage, information provision, etc., depending on the particular professional role of the helper. To assist the reader consider the kinds of relationship that may be offered to the client, we will make some use in this book of a model of supportive roles in palliative care developed by O'Berle and Davies (1990, 1992). Their work highlighted six key dimensions, which overlap significantly with the common factors which research suggests underpin effective counselling of any kind. These dimensions or ways of relating and responding to clients are:

- Valuing: having respect for the inherent worth of others regardless of particular characteristics of any one individual.
- Connecting: refers to the helper getting 'in touch' with the patient's and family members' experience. There are three aspects to connecting: making the connection, sustaining the connection, and breaking the connection.
- Empowering: enabling the patient and family to act for themselves, make their own decisions and meet their own needs. This autonomy helps maintain a sense of self-efficacy and self-worth. Empowering draws on resources that are intrinsic to the patient and family.
- Doing for: primarily directed towards and focused upon physical care. This draws on resources and skills that are extrinsic to the patient and family.
- Finding meaning: helping patients and family 'make sense' of their experience of illness, which may seem fragmented and confusing. This may include talking openly about death when the patient and their family want to do so.
- Preserving one's own integrity: maintaining feelings of self-worth and self-esteem to sustain energy and well-being. With-

out this, the helper's ability to support others becomes seriously compromised.

In order to offer sensitive support, the HCP must be able to
reflect on what kind of support is needed, not just how to offer
this. We suggest that careful consideration of the supportive roles
needed in a given situation provides a useful complement and
guide to the core counselling skills outlined previously.

Summary

- The central concern of palliative care is improving the quality
  of remaining life and the manner of dying for those who
  cannot be cured, together with supporting their family and
  friends.
- Palliative care is often associated with care in hospices, but only
  a minority of patients requiring palliative care are admitted to
  hospices. Palliative care may be provided by many different
  professionals in a wide variety of settings, including the home,
  hospitals and nursing homes.
- High quality palliative care requires effective multidisciplinary
  team work and good communication. Without this, care may
  become fragmented or else become overly intrusive, leading to
  escalating frustrations for patients, families and professionals.
- There is an extensive range of difficulties which patients and
  families dealing with a progressive life-threatening condition
  may face. These issues will partly depend on factors such as
  the specific illness involved, the family life-cycle, and local
  resources. However, life-threatening illness of any sort presents
  existential challenges of isolation, meaninglessness, choice
  and, of course, death itself.
- Research into counselling has identified some common helpful
  factors which seem to underpin most or all therapeutic work.
  These core counselling skills include:
  - working with the client's goals
  - emphasizing client's strengths, not just their difficulties
  - paying attention to the context of the problems and the pos-
    sible solutions
  - offering support through a relationship which the client

experiences as non-judgemental, genuine and offering unconditional positive regard or respect
  - helping the client to make sense of their experiences
  - helping the client to feel hope
- Research into supportive roles in palliative care has identified six key dimensions in relating to clients which may help guide our use of core counselling skills. These supportive roles are: valuing, connecting, empowering, doing for, finding meaning, preserving one's own integrity.
- Counselling skills may be offered concurrently with other forms of support depending on the particular professional role of the helper and the types of 'doing for' specific to their work.
- All counselling skills are offered through the intentional use of a supportive relationship between the self of the helper and the self of the client, involving two whole people whatever their roles and whatever the disease process involved.

Chapter 2

Joining the palliative care system

Introduction

It seems simply common sense to argue that it is vital for the palliative care of a patient to start in the right way. How we begin often sets the tone for what follows, both in terms of actions and expectations. However, in practice, it is not always easy to determine when palliative care begins.

Sometimes this is because potentially curative treatments are still under way, as when a cancer patient is living with symptoms such as lymphodoema which need palliative care, but is also receiving chemotherapy aimed at preventing any recurrence of the cancer itself. At other times, it may be clear to the professionals involved that further treatment has to be aimed at symptom relief rather than cure, but the patient (and/or other family members) has not yet understood this or seems unwilling to 'accept' this. Defining the 'start point' of palliative care may also seem problematic when events have moved so rapidly that patients and families have hardly had any opportunity to reflect on what is happening and what kind of care is needed (an extreme example is when a bad road traffic accident leads to a previously fit and healthy person being plunged into a permanent vegetative state).

In this chapter, we will discuss three examples illustrating how patients and their families may 'join' the palliative care system, and review how we, as professionals, can use counselling skills to shape helpful responses.

Case note 6

Cathy was a 26-year-old nurse who had started work at the hospice two weeks previously, after five years working mainly in medical and surgical areas. She was excited about her new job, which she had joined as she felt frustrated with staff shortages and the 'pace' and 'pressure' of busy acute settings. Cathy felt she could offer the quality of care she wanted in the hospice environment, and had taken a cut in grade to come to the hospice.

Cathy greeted Mr Jordan and his wife as they arrived at the hospice by ambulance. Mr Jordan was an elderly man transferring from a medical ward at a nearby teaching hospital, where he had been admitted after a fall at home. He had fractured his femur in four places as a result of widespread bone metastases. As the ambulance crew were taking Mr Jordan by stretcher to his bed, his wife took Cathy's arm and pulled her aside. She whispered: 'He thinks this is a rehabilitation ward – you won't tell him differently will you? It would kill him. He's always had a fear of these places and he's coping so well with his chemotherapy it would be too cruel to dash all his hopes.'

Making a connection

The foundation of effective palliative care is to find a way to connect with patients and their carers. In this instance, Cathy is offered an opportunity to form a rapid connection with Mrs Jordan by agreeing to keep secret the true nature of the hospice from Mr Jordan (and by implication to avoid discussing Mr Jordan's actual prognosis with him). Mrs Jordan's own fear and distress seem evident in her remarks, and this kind of invitation to keep a secret to protect someone can be quite seductive. Cathy may be tempted to offer immediate comfort and reassurance to

Mrs Jordan by agreeing. However, this would start the palliative care of Mr Jordan on a rather slippery slope with many attendant risks. Some of the dangers are that:

- Cathy may find herself making a promise that she cannot keep either ethically or practically. Mr Jordan might ask her directly: 'What is this place? One of the other patients said it was a hospice.' Other healthcare professionals (HCPs) may not honour a promise of secrecy made on the team's behalf by Cathy. Breaking the promise might well lead to a major rift and loss of trust between the palliative care team and Mrs Jordan, compromising and complicating future care (Bor *et al.* 1998: ch. 9).
- Cathy would be prematurely foreclosing her chances of making meaningful connections with Mr Jordan by agreeing not to discuss certain topics with him. This could lead to escalating problems if Mr Jordan's experience of his illness and the care provided were increasingly at odds with his beliefs about the care that should be provided – for example, if he becomes distressed that he is not receiving enough physiotherapy to help him walk again, or becomes angry with himself for not trying harder to make a 'better recovery'.
- Cathy might inadvertently reinforce and exacerbate some fears and fantasies that Mrs Jordan (and perhaps Mr Jordan) may already hold about hospices and palliative care. It is possible that both Mrs and Mr Jordan assume that no patients leave hospices alive, and see them simply as places to die rather than places which might help control symptoms better so that some patients may return home. Either might also be very worried that death from cancer will inevitably be unbearably painful, or by the belief that their partner 'couldn't cope with the truth'.

Clearly, these are significant risks. There could be a temptation to side-step the issues by ignoring or dismissing Mrs Jordan's plea ('I'll pass that message on to the doctor for you, Mrs Jordan', or: 'Let's just get him settled in first shall we? Can I get one of the volunteers to get you some tea?'). Such responses might well seem uncaring and unhearing. More harshly, Cathy might answer: 'Mrs Jordan, this is a hospice and we feel it's important to give patients the information they want. It all depends on what Mr Jordan wants.' The message here is that Mrs Jordan is 'in the wrong', and that the hospice is on the patient's side rather than supporting both patient and carer(s).

Thinking back to the six key dimensions of palliative care presented in Chapter 1 reminds us that the HCP in this situation needs to find a way to preserve her own integrity, to value both Mrs Jordan's needs and concerns but also Mr Jordan's, and to connect with both. There is also a need to support and empower Mrs Jordan's evident wish to shape her husband's care without disempowering Mr Jordan. Mrs Jordan's remarks also offer some early clues to the meanings which she and perhaps Mr Jordan may attribute to their experiences of his illness and treatment.

One useful response might be: 'Yes, I think you're right that many people can be quite frightened about coming to a place like this, especially if they aren't sure what kind of help we can offer. Once we've got Mr Jordan comfortable in his bed, perhaps you and I should take some time to talk in private so that you can tell us more about him and what's been happening for both of you, and I can let you know a bit more about the work that we do here.'

This reply may be useful in a number of ways. It reflects back that Cathy has heard Mrs Jordan talking about fear, while sensitively leaving open the possibility that Mrs Jordan may indirectly be talking about her own fear as much as Mr Jordan's. The response also conveys a message to Mrs Jordan that she and Mr Jordan are not alone in feeling afraid in this context ('normalization'), and that staff in the hospice are willing to hear and discuss this. The HCP's words also convey a respectful, valuing appreciation that Mrs Jordan's views are important to the staff and may help them to care for Mr Jordan. The nurse protects her own integrity by avoiding untenable promises without rebuffing Mrs Jordan's approach. Mrs Jordan is invited to help the staff (and hence herself) make some sense of what has been happening and how this contributes to the current care needs. The HCP also conveys a message that the hospice offers 'help', an active message of hope. The invitation to a more extended discussion, combined with some information giving, creates the opportunity to explore further what kind of goals Mrs Jordan feels will be important, and to consider this in combination with Mr Jordan's wishes.

Working alliances and therapeutic neutrality

In terms borrowed from family systems counselling, the aim is to connect with Mrs Jordan and eventually with Mr Jordan through a working alliance, rather than to form a coalition against Mr Jordan (Burnham 1986: 19). Coalitions are relationships where two or more people are in opposition to someone else, whereas alliances are relationships between people aimed at mutual support. Coalitions imply side-taking, alliances do not. Another way to understand this is that HCPs limit their freedom to work effectively with all those in need of care if they lose their neutrality by taking sides. Neutrality does not imply a lack of interest or coldness. The key point is that we as HCPs need to maintain our flexibility to respond to the different needs of all those involved at different times (Jones 1993: 101).

Meta-communication (communication about communication)

How we say things can be as important as what we say. Cathy's reply meta-communicates about the way in which the hospice team aims to work with patients and their families. Mrs Jordan's attempt to snatch some whispered words in the corridor may reflect previous experiences in healthcare settings where it has been difficult to gain the attention of other professionals. The HCP's words signal that staff are willing to set time aside to talk on a confidential basis with patients and carers, and also convey that the sharing of anxieties and views is an acceptable part of the treatment process rather than an 'extra' to be slipped in.

'Opening up' versus 'containing'

Other responses might be: 'I may be wrong, but it sounds like you're quite worried or frightened yourself about what's happening?' or 'What do you think he is hoping for at the moment?' or 'You say he's always been frightened of these places – what do you think he's most frightened of?'

Although these responses may well be useful at some point, they are probably less suitable for a snatched conversation in the corridor, which is not well 'boundaried' in terms of either time or private space. These questions invite Mrs Jordan to 'open up' about some potentially very upsetting topics at a moment when the HCP may not be able to offer enough uninterrupted time, privacy and attention to listen well, and may reinforce the idea that communication with nurses and other staff needs to happen 'on the move'. By contrast, the preferred intervention offers calm containment of the situation combined with an empathic response which validates Mrs Jordan's expression of concerns and gives a clear signal that there will be further opportunities to discuss them.

Good counselling skills are not simply about getting people to 'open up' about their feelings. It may also be important to help people manage and contain their feelings in some situations. Patients and relatives joining the palliative care system often feel that a lot has happened in a short space of time that has been out of their control. Sometimes there is a delicate balance to be struck between acknowledging that time may be short, without being drawn into rushing.

Case note 7

Amy is a Macmillan nurse who has been asked by the GP to make a home visit to Elaine, a single mother in her mid-thirties diagnosed with breast cancer two years previously. Shortly after diagnosis Elaine had a mastectomy, followed by a course of radiotherapy. More recently, she has been undergoing her second course of chemotherapy. The GP told Amy that Elaine is determined to get better for the sake of her two teenage daughters, and has been pushing herself to 'get fit again' and get back to her job as a part-time social worker. The GP feels that this is an unrealistic aim, and would like the Macmillan nurse to help Elaine 'make a more realistic adjustment to her illness'. Elaine has increasing breathless-ness, pain in her upper back and ribs, and continuing weight loss. Results from hospital tests suggest that she has meta-static disease which is not responding well to the chemo-therapy course. She also seems to have significant problems with nausea as a side-effect from the chemotherapy.

Amy makes contact by telephone with Elaine to arrange an initial home visit. Elaine does not seem to know that the GP has made a referral, and says very little on the telephone, but agrees that the nurse can visit her at home 'if you think you can do me any good. The GP's been pretty crap so far, though Dr Weems [oncologist coordinating the chemotherapy] has been marvellous.'

When Amy arrives, Elaine starts by saying that she doesn't see why she needs a Macmillan nurse as she's get-ting better, and criticizes her doctor angrily for being 'so pessimistic all the time, she really makes me feel ill and that's the last thing I need'. Elaine explains animatedly that she is coping very well, and has to get better as there are no other family members who could look after her daughters if 'anything happened' to her. As she talks she becomes breath-less, sweating and red in the face, and bursts into tears suddenly.

Being with a client in distress

An unhelpful response to this situation would be to accept too quickly Elaine's protestations that she doesn't need support and doesn't need a referral to the Macmillan service: 'I'm sorry I've disturbed you. I think there may have been some confusion between me and the GP.' Although Elaine has seemed dubious about the prospect of a visit by the nurse, and claims she is coping well, she has also given a number of signals ('cues') to an atten-tive listener that all is far from well. Apart from the obvious cue of crying in front of the nurse, it may also be significant that she has allowed the visit in the first place. After all, she could simply have declined a visit over the phone. Conversely, it would prob-ably be unhelpful and even downright disrespectful of the way that Elaine is trying to manage her situation to be too insistent that Elaine is not coping: 'You've been saying that you're coping really well, but I've got to say that's not how it seems right now, is it?'

The temptation to reassure patients

Many HCPs, faced with someone crying and visibly distressed, may feel an urge to try to comfort the patient. After all, this is often one of the key motivations for joining healthcare professions. A natural response to Elaine's tears might be quickly to proffer some tissues and reassurance ('Don't worry, I'm sure we can sort things out for you'), followed by an attempt at distraction, such as asking about Elaine's relationship with the doctor, or about her daughters, or the house's furnishings. While this is understandable and in some senses praiseworthy, it may not always be the most useful response for the patient in the longer term.

Assessment is a two-way process

HCPs often think about assessment as something done to patients and carers, but it is important to appreciate that patients and carers are also assessing the professionals (Lemma 1997). Whether consciously or not, the patient may be asking herself questions such as: 'Is this person someone who will listen to what I say? Will they take me seriously? Are they able to bear the sight of me in tears, or will that upset them too much?' If the Macmillan nurse immediately offers tissues and tries to comfort Elaine, this may inadvertently convey an unspoken but powerful message that Elaine's tears are unacceptable or too upsetting to Amy, and that Elaine needs to 'pull herself together' to avoid distressing the nurse.

Attentive listening

A key counselling skill is the capacity to listen attentively without interrupting clients. This includes 'listening' to non-verbal messages such as tears, as well as words. Elaine's tears are a powerful communication that all is not well.

In this situation, there have already been some clues from the referrer and from Elaine's initial comments that it has not been easy for Elaine to admit to herself and others how ill she is. While this kind of 'fighting spirit' may be an effective coping strategy for some of the time, there may also be significant drawbacks. It may also be adversely affecting her relationship with the primary care team, might block some important emotional communication with her daughters, and might mean that Elaine is continuing with treatments with unpleasant side-effects offering little benefit in symptom control. Reflecting on what has already been said, Amy could notice that even in this short time Elaine has already expressed several concerns. She is worried about how her children would manage without her support, she does not feel supported by her relationship with her GP, and she has admitted that she does 'feel ill'.

A useful initial response may be simply to sit quietly with Elaine for a while as she cries, with attention focused on her. There is of course a balance to be struck, since sitting in silence for too long may leave the client feeling abandoned or unheard. After a while, the Macmillan nurse might say something like: 'It's important to cry sometimes' (a simple validating and normalizing message), or perhaps: 'It seems like there are a lot of tears ready to pour out now. I wonder, have your daughters seen you like this, or is it something that you usually try to keep from them?' This intervention gives genuine or 'congruent' feedback that the nurse hears the depth of the distress. It also offers an acknowledgement that Elaine's status as a responsible mother may be very significant in the way that she feels she needs to deal with the experience of having cancer. The wording also carries a broader message (a meta-communication) that palliative care staff such as the Macmillan team are interested in talking with the client as a person in their social and family context, not simply as a patient with a physical condition to be treated.

Using touch as a way to connect

Sometimes when a client is crying and in deep distress it can be appropriate to connect with the client by offering a physical contact like a hand to be held. However, physical contact and touch need to be used very cautiously and sensitively, particularly in early encounters with a client. Here, the Macmillan nurse knows very little of Elaine's personal history and personality, and it would be very hard to gauge how 'safe' or how intrusive Elaine might find such physical contact. Generally, it is better to err on the side of caution and restraint in using touch.

Case note 8

Mr Skol was a 67-year-old man with bone and liver metastases from an unknown primary tumour, admitted to the hospice for terminal care. He was confused and very weak. He spent most of his time lying quietly in his bed at the hospice gazing at the ceiling, but sometimes asked where he was and what he was doing in a prison. He was at his most alert and lucid when his son Aaron visited him each day, when he seemed to understand that he was ill and in a 'hospital'. He appeared to enjoy these visits. Staff knew relatively little about Mr Skol's family background, except that he was widowed many years before and had four children, of whom only Aaron lived locally.

The nursing and medical staff had little contact with Aaron, who tended to slip in and out of the wards of the hospice quietly. However, the Volunteer Coordinator of the hospice began to notice that volunteer staff working in the reception area and coffee-room near the entrance to the hospice were spending increasing amounts of time in lengthy conversations with Aaron, which seemed to leave both Aaron and the volunteers visibly distressed. The volunteers explained to the Coordinator that Aaron was very frightened indeed about the prospect of his father dying, and kept saying that he didn't know how he was going to cope or what would happen when his father died. The volunteers said they tried to spend time listening to his concerns, but felt increasingly out of their depth and at a loss.

The Volunteer Coordinator spent time in the reception area next afternoon around the time Aaron usually visited.

Aaron soon began a conversation with her. He kept repeating that he was losing his home with his father dying, and said that he couldn't stop thinking about this and about how poor he would be. He complained that although he prayed every night to save his father, he had received no answer and he was becoming increasingly angry about how God had abandoned his father and all the poor and sick people in the world. As he spoke he became increasingly angry and agitated, saying: 'It's hopeless, there's no God, God is dead and my father is dying, it's all ending, it's all going to end.'

Helping family members to join or connect with the palliative care system

Palliative care aims to offer holistic support, with the family or significant social network as the focus of care, rather than simply treating the physical condition or caring for the individual patient in isolation. Although Mr Skol's care was not creating problems for the nursing and medical team, the alert Volunteer Coordinator noticed that her volunteers were becoming increasingly embroiled with Mr Skol's son to an unusual degree. We cannot assume that patients and family members will all 'join' with us at the same time or in the same way. Some people may need more time to develop confidence in using support from HCPs. In some cases, as with Aaron, HCPs may need to be observant and quite proactive in helping people make effective connections with the system.

Recognizing limits and involving others

We have already discussed how the preservation and protection of personal integrity is an important counselling skill for palliative care workers. Good palliative care relies on the combined effort of a team, rather than the heroic efforts of one worker alone. Implicit in this is the need for different members of the team to monitor each other's needs and stresses as well as their own personal stress and that of the patient. The Coordinator was sensitive to the needs of her volunteers, and made a proactive move to connect with Aaron herself, to make an assessment of his needs and the support that might be required.

In this situation the Coordinator needs to respond in a way that is containing, and that also helps assess what kinds of support Aaron could use. This requires a clarification of Aaron's hopes and fears by the purposeful use of questions as a part of risk assessment. For example, the Volunteer Coordinator might ask Aaron to talk further in a more private side-room, and ask: 'Aaron, you said that it's all going to end . . . I'm not sure what you mean by that, could you tell me a bit more about that?' If Aaron answers this in an apparently bizarre or extreme form by saying something like: 'It feels like the world is coming to an end – there will be no sun, and time will stop', this would be a strong indication that the hospice staff may need to arrange support for Aaron from more specialist psychiatric services, given the apparent disconnection between Aaron's experience and objective reality, indicative of a psychotic episode.

It is of course possible that such difficulties are part of a longer-standing pattern, and so it may also be helpful to ask questions about the historical context of these kind of ideas and distress: 'Are there times that you've felt like this before?' Questions such as: 'Aaron, have you talked about these kinds of worries before with anyone? Who was that? Are you in contact with them now, or do you think it might be helpful for us to help you get in contact with them again?' may help clarify whether Aaron is already known to mental health services.

Referring on can be an important professional skill, not a weakness

All healthcare staff need to understand that effective assessment leading to the involvement of other services is a useful skill, not a sign of failure on the part of the HCP making the initial contact. Involving specialist mental health services in this way need not mean that the hospice team have no further role in supporting Aaron, but does mean that advice can be taken about appropriate responses and involvement, rather than leaving volunteer staff struggling to respond to someone experiencing severe mental illness.

It may be instead that Aaron's answer is less bizarre but still gives the Volunteer Coordinator reason to be concerned about Aaron's safety (or indeed the safety of others). For example, Aaron might say: 'I don't know really, I just feel like it's all going to end soon – I don't think I can go on after my father's died, I've lived with him all my life, I wouldn't know how to cope on my own.'

Sometimes HCPs worry that by asking about the risk of self-harm or suicide, they may 'put ideas into someone's head', in other words increase the risk by asking about it. In fact, research suggests the opposite (Russell and Hersov 1983). Allowing people an opportunity to share such ideas and fears may actually be therapeutic in its own right, as a frightening, possibly shameful secret thought is shared with another who does not shy away.

Additionally, encouraging disclosure of thoughts about harm to oneself (or to others) creates possibilities for involving people and services which can help monitor and protect from these risks, whether this be the vigilance of other family members, professional support from a counsellor or community psychiatric nurse, or anti-depressant treatment. It is an important counselling skill to be able to ask questions about potentially frightening topics which other people may have been unable or unwilling to ask.

Main learning points

- The way that care starts often sets the tone for what follows. This may be complicated since the starting point for palliative care may be unclear or seem different for different people.
- Good quality care requires us to form meaningful personal connections with patients and their families. This responsibility is shared by all members of the palliative care team.
- We must ensure that connections with one person are not made at the expense of relationships with other family members. Working alliances between people are healthier than coalitions against others.

- When patients join palliative care, the anxiety of change may create pressure to sort out many things at once. Take time and space to gather your thoughts and composure.
- Ensure that the client feels they have been listened to and understood. This may be achieved verbally, but can also be conveyed through non-verbal communication and your 'presence' with the person.
- Effective counselling skills need not mean deep conversations or encouraging patients to 'open up'. Facilitating containment of feelings and emotions may be equally important.
- Assessment is a two-way process. Patients and relatives are assessing us and our capacities, at the same time as we try to understand them and their needs.

Chapter 3

Empowering patients, finding goals and resources

Introduction

When someone close to us is ill, it is a very ordinary and compassionate reaction to try to look after them, to do things for them, to offer 'care' (Benner and Wrubel 1989). This helps us to feel useful, and provides a means for us to show our love. Many of us would recognize the attractions of being comforted and tended to when we are ill ourselves. However, problems may arise in palliative care when the patient is 'cared for' to the exclusion of other forms of interaction, or when the need of the carer(s) to offer care begins to predominate over the wishes and interests of the patient (Ellis 1997).

Palliative care staff often have to walk a fine line between providing care to patients and helping patients continue to care for themselves. HCPs need to strike a balance between being sensitively responsive to patient need and disempowering patients, leaving them little space in their own care except for the adoption of a 'sick role'.

In this chapter, we use three examples to review ways in which counselling skills can help clarify care needs without disempowering.

Case note 9

Matthew had been an independent and proud man throughout his adult life. With a childhood spent mainly in orphanages and children's homes, he had learnt to 'stand on his own two feet'. He had never married or had children, but had enjoyed a busy working life as a plumber in a small firm over several decades, with many friends from work and the local allotment society.

Matthew had haemophilia and needed clotting factor blood products throughout his life. At the age of 54 he suffered episodes of nausea and diarrhoea, began to lose weight, and developed painful skin lesions on his legs. Matthew was diagnosed as having AIDS, probably contracted from HIV-contaminated blood products. He started combination drug therapy, but responded poorly to this. The skin lesions proliferated, and Matthew suffered increasing problems with painful swollen legs and related walking difficulties. Matthew was admitted to a palliative care unit from his home for review of pain control and treatment of the lymphodoema in his legs.

Treatment seemed to progress well, and Matthew was a 'popular' patient who seemed to relate well to staff and other patients. However, Matthew grew quiet and moody when senior staff tried to discuss plans for sending him home again. He began to complain of renewed problems with pain control, and slept poorly, frequently calling night staff to sit by him in the small hours. One such night he started complaining bitterly to Francis, an auxiliary nurse, that he felt useless and frightened. He realized that doctors at the hospice felt he was 'swinging the lead' and should go home again, but he felt that he was incapable of looking after himself any more. He was so relieved to be in a place where staff were on hand to take care of him 'in case anything happens', and to keep him from becoming lonely.

Empathic acknowledgement

Listening empathically to the feelings expressed (rather than the detail of the content), Francis will hear that Matthew is frightened, lonely, worrying about the future, feeling useless. Another theme may be anger. One of the most basic tasks in this situation is simply but importantly to help Matthew feel that he has been heard and understood, at least to a degree. This is especially important since part of Matthew's complaint is that other people do not seem to believe him or fully appreciate the difficulty of his situation. It is not enough for Francis to understand Matthew's concerns empathically. For this encounter to be therapeutic, the auxiliary nurse must also help Matthew know that his communication has been understood and valued, that there is a genuine attempt to understand him as a valued person.

Patronizing reassurance/dismissing concerns

It would probably be unhelpful for Francis to respond to Matthew's concerns simply by reassuring or 'pacifying' him, by arguing that his concerns are ill-founded: 'Oh, Matthew, don't be silly. I'm sure the doctors don't think you're swinging the lead,' or: 'You're doing yourself down there Matthew – you've been getting on ever so well and I'm sure you'll be able to manage better than you expect at home.' Although there might be some degree of 'objective' truth to both statements, neither are congruent with Matthew's current experience and emotions.

Equally, it would be inappropriate for Francis to pass off Matthew's remarks with a joke ('Lonely without us? Goodness, I'd have thought you'll be glad to see the last of our motley crew!'), or to sidestep the conversation entirely: 'Oh, dear, this is the second night in a row you've had problems sleeping. Do you want some sleeping pills?' Matthew is likely to feel misunderstood and perhaps patronized. He may decide there is no point trying to talk about these feelings again. He may become even more frightened and anxious about the future. If a patient has an illness they know to be progressive and which causes pain, and they begin to believe that others do not believe they are suffering, they may worry how much others will respond if their symptoms recur or worsen.

Avoid premature closure

Francis may assume too quickly that he understands what Matthew means. Although Matthew has volunteered some strong cues, the meaning of these for Matthew is not self-evident. If Matthew is angry, what is he most angry at? If Matthew is feeling 'useless', is this to do with feeling out of control and unable to 'fix things up' as he has through his working life (self-efficacy), or he is meaning more that he feels unimportant and worthless (self-esteem)?

Hypothesizing and curiosity

Two different counselling skills are relevant here for the HCP. One is the capacity to *hypothesize*. That is, to imagine possible explanations and meanings linked with the patient's experience and their account. What reasons might Matthew have to be angry or frightened? Why might Matthew doubt the competence or caring of doctors? The other is the capacity to remain *curious*. That is, to assume that there is always more to understand. Staying curious helps the HCP avoid becoming too attached to their interpretations of patients' words and behaviour (Cecchin 1987). Although Francis might hypothesize that Matthew may have good reason to mistrust doctors because of his accidental HIV infection, this may not be a factor at all. Although Francis might hypothesize that Matthew's institutionalized childhood has left him with very mixed feelings about having to depend on others, this might not be significant for Matthew.

   Francis may begin by responding simply: 'I'm sorry that you're so upset at the moment. I think a lot of patients do get frightened and lonely at times like this, that's very natural. Would you like me to stay so that we can talk about that some more now, or shall I let you rest again?' This offers an empathic acknowledgement of the loneliness and fear, validating these as emotions that can be talked about with staff, and normalizing them as emotions that many people with illness have.

Offering choice

This way of responding offers a genuine invitation to continue the conversation further, but leaving Matthew with choice over whether and when to continue. Taking such conversations step by step and checking whether the patient wants to go further at each stage is in itself a form of patient empowerment, offering an antidote to professional curiosity and a 'need to know' for the HCP's benefit rather than the patient's (Ellis 1997). Note how this kind of invitation offers much greater choice than: 'I'm sorry that you're so upset at the moment. We could talk about that tomorrow if you want,' or: 'Shall I ask the counsellor to speak with you tomorrow about that?', both of which prevent Matthew opting to speak with Francis there and then.

Inviting a continuation

If Matthew does choose to continue the conversation, it may be useful for the HCP to pause and wait to see how Matthew would like to continue. The patient has mentioned a variety of feelings and concerns, and the HCP should avoid second-guessing which of these is most significant to Matthew. However, if Matthew seems very unsure how to continue, the HCP might invite Matthew to say more about one of the emotionally charged terms he has used. For example: 'I think you said something about "in case anything happens". I wondered what you meant?', or: 'You said you felt "useless and frightened" sometimes. Could you say more about that?' or simply: 'It sounds like you've got a lot on your mind at the moment. What's bothering you most?'

Ending the contact

When Matthew chooses to discontinue the conversation, the HCP might make a point of saying: 'Please do call me if you would like to talk again, or if you need anything else.' This reaffirms the acceptability of such contacts and disclosures, while also leaving open the possibility that Matthew might also need other assistance (such as analgesia, toileting, etc.). The use of counselling skills to manage therapeutic conversations about distress should complement and integrate with the physical/biomedical needs of palliative care patients. Talking about his situation may in time offer some relief to Matthew but this does not preclude use of medication as well.

Attending to the broader context(s)

Thinking about the broader context for this night-time conversation between a frightened patient and junior staff member, Francis would perhaps be mindful that Matthew may be rather angry with himself for not coping 'better' and perhaps ashamed of this, given his upbringing and independent adult life. Francis might also wonder whether Matthew's childhood in orphanages and homes has left him rather wary of challenging or directly expressing feelings of vulnerability to authority figures (such as senior hospice staff trying to discuss discharge plans with him). There may be value in supporting Matthew to communicate more openly with other hospice staff, particularly in view of the potential stalemate about discharge planning that is developing.

Colluding against other staff versus promoting conversations with others

One pitfall would be to collude with Matthew's complaints about the sceptical attitude of other hospice staff by siding with him against them (sympathizing rather than empathizing): 'Oh, I know what you mean. I get so annoyed with them when they try to discharge patients like you too soon. That happened last week with another patient I knew, and he had to come straight back in the next day.' While this might briefly help Matthew feel less alone, this would not facilitate clearer communication between him and other staff, and would leave him with a feeling that the care team is divided or split.

The way in which Francis talks with Matthew about these issues may help Matthew practise ways of explaining himself to others, and help him gauge how HCPs may respond to his feelings. This conversation with a junior staff member may thus be therapeutic in its own right, and also help empower Matthew to take risks in disclosing his concerns to others. As he begins to do this, the palliative care team will find it easier to explore what his goals are and negotiate support. For example, reducing loneliness may be a more significant goal for Matthew than returning home, yet with sensitive support (e.g. day-care attendance) these may not be incompatible goals.

As the conversations unfolds, asking simple questions such as: 'How much of this have you told the doctors so far?' or: 'Who else do you think needs to know about these concerns of yours so we can try to get things right for you? How will you go about letting them know?' would raise for discussion Matthew's role and responsibility in helping staff plan his care. This approach is more open-ended and empowering than simply telling Matthew: 'You really must talk with the social worker about this. If they don't know, they can't help you.'

Case note 10

Pip was determined not to 'give in' to her breast cancer. Despite increasing problems with breathlessness and two recent rib fractures, she was determined to take part in a fund-raising walk to Land's End being organized by her local complementary health centre. She was encouraged in this by her faith healer, Thomas, who held regular 'visualization' sessions at the health centre for cancer patients at which they were exhorted to maintain a fighting spirit, and turn this against the cancerous cells in their body like a 'spiritual laser'. Pip had a good relationship with her GP who was pleased that she was 'keeping her spirits up'.

   Pip's long-term partner Alessandra took Emma, the district nurse, to one side on a home visit. She asked Emma to try to persuade Pip not to go on the trip. Alessandra explained that she was concerned both for Pip's well-being and also for their two young children, Lisa and Averil. She felt that Pip was 'in denial' about the extent of her illness and needlessly putting herself at risk of further fractures and exhaustion. Alessandra said that the children were already very worried about their mother and having problems sleeping, and she thought it would be too hard on them if their mother stayed away overnight at a time like this.

Coping strategies

One of the tensions inherent in respecting the needs of carers as well as patients themselves, is that different people in the caring system will have different concerns, may not agree about goals and may prefer to adopt quite different coping strategies. Some strategies focus on action and problem-solving, while others may be more emotion-focused (Lazarus and Folkman 1984). Following Stroebe and Stroebe (1995: 203) coping strategies may include:

- confrontive coping (e.g. letting feelings 'out', fighting for what you want – fighting spirit);
- distancing (e.g. trying not to think about the situation);
- self-controlling (e.g. trying to keep your feelings to yourself, and carrying on 'as normal');
- seeking social support (e.g. asking others for advice, sharing feelings with others);
- accepting responsibility (e.g. self-criticism, promising to do things differently 'next time');
- escape-avoidance (e.g. hoping for miracles, fantasizing, comfort eating, smoking);
- planful problem solving (e.g. making plans, changing lifestyle);
- positive reappraisal (e.g. reconsidering 'what really matters', finding faith, growing 'as a person')

Are coping strategies useful?

These coping strategies are potentially some of the major psychological resources that people have to draw on in times of stress. However, they may or may not be successful in helping someone to manage or live with a stressful situation or an illness. The utility of any given strategy is likely to vary with factors such as:

- the nature of the problem (e.g. distancing oneself from symptoms of an undiagnosed but treatable cancer may have quite different implications from distancing oneself from symptoms of a diagnosed and inoperable cancer);

- the beliefs and personal style of the person trying to cope;
- the beliefs and style of other significant people in the situation;
- the degree of effort needed to keep up the strategy.

In practice, people often use a combination of coping strategies, with the balance between these changing over time and across situations.

In situations such as that presented, it can be useful for the HCP to hypothesize (develop some possible explanations) about the reason for the request as one way to try to understand and empathize with the person seeking support. Alessandra's request for help alerts Emma to an apparent 'mis-fit' between the coping strategies currently being used by Pip and those preferred by her partner:

- When Alessandra describes her partner as being 'in denial', this may represent some mix of confrontive coping (challenging the limitations the illness imposes), distancing (minimizing the extent of her disease, whether consciously or not), and seeking social support (from the self-help group). It is quite possible that Pip might describe her attitude as fighting spirit rather than denial.
- By contrast, Alessandra seems to be seeking social support (from the district nurse) and trying planful problem solving (how to look after the children). Emma might also wonder whether, in expressing concerns about the children, Alessandra is also distancing or trying to keep hidden (self-controlling) some of her own feelings about her partner's illness.

Self-reflexivity and a non-judgemental attitude

As HCPs we need to reflect carefully on our own assumptions and beliefs about coping with illness (Nordman *et al.* 1998). If we can monitor our own feelings and biases, this may help us to remain non-judgemental in relation to the problem presented. If Emma is especially sensitive to the emotional vulnerability of children being left without their mother (for example, if her own children are a similar age) she may have to work hard to avoid siding strongly with Alessandra against Pip from the beginning ('Poor children. They need their mother more than ever at a time like this, I'd be happy to talk with Pip about that. I wonder if she knows what effect all this is having on them?'). Conversely, if Emma believes that 'fighting spirit' is a particularly good way of coping with cancer (perhaps if she has already 'beaten' cancer herself a few years ago), she may have to be particularly careful not to inadvertently leave Alessandra feeling unheard ('I appreciate that you're worried, but perhaps this is just Pip's way of coping with things. Different people find different things helpful').

We are not arguing for or against a particular combination of coping strategies to be used by Pip and Alessandra. The task for the HCP is not to impose her own judgement, but to help others articulate and reflect on their own strategies, and how well these mesh with the strategies of others involved.

The challenge for Emma is to respond in a way which genuinely validates Alessandra's feelings and allows opportunities for further discussion, but remaining neutral rather than taking sides. Therapeutic neutrality should not mean coldness. Rather, it means maintaining balanced relationships with the significant people in a system and retaining flexibility about interventions and action in the future. Taking sides with Alessandra might have significant adverse consequences for Emma's relationship with Pip, and perhaps also with the GP and other members of the cancer self-help group. If Emma replies simply: 'I haven't really got a view on that – it's something for you and her to discuss together', this might well seem very uncaring and unhelpful.

More constructively, the district nurse might reply: 'Thank you for letting me know about Lisa and Averil. I hadn't realized they were having trouble sleeping. I suppose an illness like this can be hard on everyone. What has Pip said when you've talked about this with her?' This acknowledges Pip's illness as something of shared concern. Emma validates Alessandra's approach, and invites Alessandra to reflect on her own responsibility in tackling the issue rather than taking this on for her.

Suppose Alessandra were to reply: 'Well, I know she feels very strongly about going, and I thought it might sound better coming from you,' the HCP could continue by asking: 'Suppose for a moment you did try to discuss it with Pip – how would you put it to her?' The intention is to support Alessandra to articulate her concerns and plan for a possible discussion with Pip.

Case note 11

Eric was the youngest of Edwin and Michaela's children. At the age of 19 he was still living at home with his parents, but was applying for City and Guilds courses and hoping to become an electrician like his father. He had begun to save some money towards a 'moving out' fund from casual jobs. He and his girlfriend Marsha dreamt of getting a flat together, although neither of their families supported this idea.

Eric began to develop balance problems and muscle weakness, and seemed to become withdrawn and rather depressed, which surprised his family as he had always been very outgoing. These problems worsened, and eventually the family was offered a provisional diagnosis of new variant CJD (Creutzfeld-Jakob disease).

The family felt devastated. Marsha broke off her relationship with Eric and stopped visiting altogether. As Eric increasingly remained in bed and grew increasingly inarticulate, his father started staying out drinking in the evenings more and more, while his mother abandoned her own part-time college teaching to stay in looking after Eric. After a while, she moved a folding bed into his room and started sleeping alongside him.

The GP knew the family well, and was understandably upset and concerned at the illness itself, but was also increasingly concerned about the split developing between Edwin and Michaela, and the apparent lack of communication in the household.

Using counselling skills to offer support proactively

Using counselling skills well is not simply a matter of reacting to things that other people have already said. Counselling skills may also help the healthcare professional (HCP) develop hypotheses about a clinical situation which suggest ways to offer support proactively. This can be seen as connecting by reaching out, rather than simply accepting an approach. It may be importan to notice conversations which are *not* happening, or things whic seem to remain unspoken, so that the HCP can try to empow family members to talk together in new ways.

The psychosocial typology of disease

The impact of a disease on a patient and family is not simp. to do with its physical effects. We must take into account th psychological and social aspects of conditions ('psychosoci. typology' – Rolland 1994: ch. 2). Important psychosocial aspec might include:

- how 'shameful' or stigmatizing the condition is (e.g. AID versus heart disease);
- whether or not the disease is linked to certain lifestyle choic((e.g. prostate cancer versus lung cancer);
- whether the disease affects communication and/or cognitiv skills (e.g. stomach cancer versus brain tumour);
- whether others will worry if the disease is contagious or ma be inherited;
- whether the outcome of the disease is certain or unknown (e.; CJD versus breast cancer);
- whether the disease is visible to others or hidden;
- whether the family has dealt with similar illnesses before;
- whether the disease produces continuous or intermitter symptoms.

In this instance, the GP would be aware that CJD is a rar and relatively new disease. Family members may have few model from their own experience or from popular culture of how t 'deal' with such illness, and are unlikely to know other familie who have been through a similar experience. There may be rela tively few support structures and organizations compared witl more common illnesses such as diabetes or cancer. Adding to th psychosocial strain that this rarity poses, CJD is currently know as an irreversible, untreatable and incurable disease leading t death via distressing symptoms, including major cognitive an communication impairments.

The relationship between illness and the family life-cycle

Attending to the family structure reminds us that the illness has cut across or even reversed many 'normal' developmental processes in the family life-cycle (Rolland 1994; Carter and McGoldrick 1999). At a time when the family might have been expecting Edwin to be moving on into adulthood and healthily separating from his family of origin, his illness and care needs have rendered him highly dependent for even basic physical care.

The illness is traumatic not simply because of its symptomatology and the potential of an 'untimely' death (in this instance, a child dying before his parents), but has also occurred at a time when considerable change was underway in the family balance. The CJD has raised new demands at a point when Edwin and Michaela might have been anticipating the pleasure and/or challenge of renegotiating their own relationship as a couple in their own right, and may have been developing new plans for their individual careers.

Perhaps the GP should do nothing?

Of course, one option in this case is for the GP simply to notice their own distress, but choose to wait for the family to offer a cue for further discussions. However, the pattern which the GP can see developing is one of non-communication in a deteriorating condition of high psychosocial burden, and early intervention may be valuable. The challenge is to do this in a way that is experienced as supportive and unthreatening.

Some unhelpful ways of responding

The couple might well feel at fault if the GP raised the subject during a home visit by saying something like: 'I've noticed that the two of you don't seem to be getting on very well together these days. I realize you're under a lot of strain, but I wondered if we needed to think about getting things right between you two so we're all pulling in the same direction?'

Similarly, if the GP met with Michaela on a visit while Edwin was out and commented: 'Oh, is Edwin out again? I wondered if we needed to get together to talk about that, to make sure that you're getting enough support', this could (i) reinforce hostile feelings Michaela may be harbouring about her husband's absence, (ii) make Michaela feel defensive in response to the implicit criticism of her husband, and (iii) reinforce an unspoken assumption that Michaela should naturally be the primary carer for Eric whether she feels able to continue this role in the longer term or not.

A third form of problematic response might be: 'I realize that an illness like this puts you both under considerable strain, so I'd like to refer you both to our practice counsellor who'd be able to offer you some sessions as a couple.' Although the issues involved are complex, and skilled couple counselling might indeed be a helpful support, the referral itself needs to be negotiated and understood as a support rather than criticism.

More helpfully

More helpfully, the GP might try to open a conversation with the couple during a home visit by suggesting: 'I've been thinking about all of you quite a bit recently. The more I think about it, the more I realize what a distressing situation it is for a family for someone so young as Eric to have an illness like this. I hope you don't mind my asking, but I wanted to ask a few questions about how you've been dealing with things as a family. Would that be OK?' The remark is congruent and open, and frames the issue as a family-illness one, rather than a couple problem.

The couple may decline

Although the remark clearly invites further conversation, the GP begins slowly, offering Edwin and Michaela a chance to decline. If they replied: 'Well, actually, I think we're doing OK. It's kind of you to ask, but I'd rather not get into that side of things right now', the GP might conclude by respecting this while leaving the door open for future discussions: 'OK, that's fine. Do remember, I'm here for both of you as well, not just for Eric, so let me know if there is anything I can help with.' The GP respects the couple's autonomy while reaffirming his or her availability as a family resource and the validity of discussing family issues, not just symptoms. It would be inappropriate to push the matter further at this point, especially since the conversation was initiated by the GP rather than linking from cues expressed by the couple.

One partner may decline while the other wishes to speak

One partner might decline: 'Actually Doc, I think we're doing OK, thanks anyway,' while the other partner disagrees (e.g. snorting and shaking their head as the other speaks, or: 'Well, you may be fine, but I'm not'). The GP may proceed simply by commenting: 'You feel the family's coping OK at present, but I think you're [turning to the other] saying you're not so sure? Could you say a bit more about that?' The GP may be performing a useful role in helping the couple to tolerate the tension of airing different views about the situation, and validating the expression of concerns, without taking sides with one partner or the other.

In this instance the GP would need to proceed with careful neutrality, alternating discussion with one partner by checking perceptions with the other ('Edwin's saying that (x) worries him, but I appreciate that you may feel differently about some things. What's your view of (x)?').

If it becomes clear that one person would like to talk further while the other continues to prefer to keep a lid on things, the GP might suggest: 'I appreciate that you may have different ways of dealing with this situation. If either of you would like to talk further with me, I'd be happy to make more time to do that at the surgery. Do let me know if you'd like that.' Trying to continue the conversation with the couple jointly at this time runs the risk of antagonizing the partner who would rather not talk, and may prejudice future relationships.

The couple agree to allow the GP to ask some questions

If the couple agree to let the GP ask some questions about the family functioning, some useful ways to begin might include:

'I guess this illness has been hard on all of you, but I wondered who in the family has been most affected besides Eric?', and then: 'Why do you think that's so?'

'I was wondering what you find most difficult about the illness – and I suppose the answer may be different for each of you. Edwin, what's hardest for you? Michaela, what's hardest for you?'

Coping questions

Coping questions (George *et al.* 1990) like: 'What's been helping you to cope with that so far?' and: 'How has [your partner] been helping you to deal with that?' may be useful ways to acknowledge the difficulties, but also to help bring to light coping strategies and resources in the family. First, it may be useful for family members to develop a more explicit awareness of what does help. Second, it may be helpful for family members to hear what others appreciate about their efforts. Third, these kinds of questions will help assess whether there are current dilemmas where there are few or no effective coping strategies, clarifying where further intervention may be needed.

Given that the GP is partly motivated by a concern about the relationship between the couple, it may also be helpful to ask questions which invite the partners to empathize with the position of the other: 'Looking ahead a little bit, what do you think Edwin may find most difficult as Eric becomes less well? How do you think he might deal with that?' The point is not so much to secure answers there and then, but rather to help the couple begin to ask themselves these questions and share some discussion about them. A broader message is also communicated, that these are aspects of care about which the GP could validly be consulted.

The emphasis at this stage is not about offering expert advice; rather, the GP aims to:

- empower the couple to begin to talk about the family dynamics if they wish, legitimizing discussion of psychosocial and family themes as well as discussion of biomedical aspects of care;
- help the couple to notice and take credit for what they are already doing which is helpful;
- help the couple and the GP develop an awareness and capacity to discuss aspects of family functioning which are causing distress and which need further attention.

The GP need not feel overwhelmed by a responsibility to follow up all these aspects in much greater depth. Part of the aim is to help the couple begin to communicate in this way, and part of the aim is to assess whether the couple find it helpful to talk in this way. At the end of the meeting the GP may ask: 'Thanks for taking the time to answer my questions. I wanted to ask whether you'd found it useful spending some time together thinking through these things a little?' If the couple respond positively, this may be the time to suggest: 'We do have a counsellor based at our practice. Of course I'll be seeing you and Eric again, and I'm happy to talk some more about the family issues if that'd be helpful, but I also wondered if you might be interested in meeting with the practice counsellor?'

Main learning points

- Caring for others who are ill is an important motivation for most healthcare workers. However, to avoid disempowering patients and relatives we must also focus on helping people continue to care for themselves.
- Empathizing with patients helps us understand what their goals and concerns might be. Empathic acknowledgement should be offered back to them, providing feedback about their attempts to communicate, and chances to correct us.
- Offering premature or false reassurance is unhelpful and disempowering. It may inhibit the expression of further concerns, foster unrealistic expectations and undermine trust.
- Validating and normalizing patients' concerns may facilitate further expression. This may include providing 'permission'

or support to discuss feared topics which are otherwise avoided.

- Many patients with serious illnesses have experienced significant losses of choice and control. Providing genuine choices, even about minor aspects of care, is a way of restoring autonomy.
- Hypothesizing is an important counselling skill, which involves the development of 'informed guesses' to guide further exploration and interventions. Hypotheses should take into account the interaction between the particular kind of illness (its psychosocial typology), the stage of the individual and family's life-cycle, and the patient's personal style and experiences.
- Maintaining curiosity about patients helps us remain open to feedback that our hypotheses need changing, and reminds us to look for the resources and coping strategies that patients have already been able to use.
- Some of the most important resources that patients have are their psychological coping strategies. These may or may not be effective in relieving distress or fit well with the coping strategies of HCPs and relatives.
- HCPs need to remain non-judgemental in relation to these strategies, while supporting patients to reflect on their utility. Self-reflection about one's beliefs and actions can help the HCP to remain non-judgemental.
- Maintaining therapeutic neutrality is important when dealing with couples and families who may have different beliefs about their problems.

Chapter 4

Living with loss

Introduction

One of the most powerful themes pervading palliative care is that of loss. As healthcare professionals (HCPs), we need to develop our sensitivity to many different kinds of loss. Our capacity to empathize and offer support will be limited by the losses that we can bring ourselves to acknowledge.

Some losses may have a physical basis linked with disease and/or treatment. Other kinds of loss may be more related to changes in relationships and beliefs. Some losses may already have occurred, while others may be anticipated but no less painful. We must also remember that any particular 'type' of loss may hold different meanings for different individuals.

In this chapter, we discuss three examples, each of which involves several different kinds of loss. In each case, the HCP must steer a difficult course between providing support and hope, without offering false reassurance or minimizing the awful nature of the losses.

Case note 12

Yolande was a 45-year-old woman with motor neurone disease. The course of her illness had been quite rapid; she had been diagnosed some three months previously when she had begun to develop some balance problems and difficulties grasping small objects with her fingers. Since then, she developed problems breathing freely, and progressively lost strength and control in all four limbs. She was admitted to the hospice when she 'went off her legs', losing her independent mobility, at the same time as her husband Sam, who was 58 years old, had a small heart attack leading to his hospitalization. She had been admitted to the hospice to provide a period of respite and assessment while her husband was treated, with the aim of discharging her home again once a suitable package of care could be arranged.

Yolande arrived in a very distressed and disoriented state, but seemed to calm down rapidly after her admission to the hospice. She spent most of her waking hours watching the television in her room, and seemed reluctant to talk about plans for discharge back home. On her fifth day in the hospice she was very abrupt with the occupational therapist who was trying to assess her skills for self-care, shouting: 'Just stop bothering me, you know I can't do anything now, I'm fine here, just go away.'

Shortly afterwards one of the nursing auxiliaries came to help her wash. As this was coming to its end, Yolande said to the auxiliary: 'I wonder if you could tell that nice young girl I'm sorry, I'm just feeling very down today and I don't really feel up to thinking about going home. I don't really want to see her again. I don't think Sam could cope with it, and I'm better off here. Please leave the door open as you go, it's such a small room here, I just feel like the walls are closing in all the time, especially at night. Please leave the door open, I want to be able to see people going past.'

Responding to patients when they need us

Practising patient-centred care, rather than professional-led care, requires us to listen carefully to the cues that patients offer us about their needs and concerns. Moreover, it requires us to pay respectful attention to the opportunities that patients use to communicate and seek support, and to respond to these flexibly rather than try to constrain patients to communicate at times and situations of our own choosing. This is one reason why all members of the palliative care team benefit from the development of good counselling skills.

Personal care as a bridge to building trust

As many nursing auxiliaries are well aware, many patients share some of their deeper feelings and fears in the context of intimate personal care and the relative 'informality' of interactions with junior staff, contrasted with more formal assessment sessions and reviews with doctors, occupational therapists, counsellors and senior nurses. For some patients, skilled and sensitive physical care can be an important channel through which they can begin to feel connected to and valued by staff (Lawler 1991). As they develop a measure of trust they may in turn risk some personal disclosure of vulnerabilities.

Responding at an inappropriate level

In this example, Yolande offers a very rich set of communications to the nursing auxiliary, in a much more invitational way than was offered to the occupational therapist. An unhelpful response would be a brief assent to the overt content of the patient's request: 'OK, Yolande, I'll make sure I pass that message on. I'm sure she'll understand. Door open, did you say? Give me a buzz if you need anything else.' Although this complies with the patient's request for action ('Doing for'), this response does not 'fit' with the emotional level that Yolande offers. It also squanders an opportunity to help acknowledge and validate her feelings ('Valuing') and perhaps explore further her experience of her illness ('Making meaning'). Offering these dimensions of care may in turn facilitate the aspects of 'empowerment' and 'doing for' that the occupational therapist was trying to provide.

Blocking the communication

There might be a temptation at some level to respond very matter-of-factly to Yolande's comments precisely because of the richness of her communication. This relatively young patient is suffering a rapid progression of a very disabling disease which has already resulted in significant disability, overlapping with her partner's serious illness and her related concerns about his own prospects. Yolande's remarks about the walls closing in may reflect distress at the loss of mobility and independence she has already suffered (in a sense, her world is indeed getting smaller because of the illness) and hinting at fears about losses yet to come including the possibility of dying through asphyxiation (Bright 1998). Her apparent fear of being left alone may relate to this kind of death anxiety. If the nursing auxiliary is feeling fragile or tired herself for any reason, or is perhaps anxious to get away and off-shift, there may be a temptation to 'block' deeper discussion. As HCPs it is important for us to find ways to look after ourselves and preserve our own integrity in palliative care, but this should not be at the expense of attending meaningfully to patients.

Broadening the focus to relationships

If the nursing auxiliary is able to offer a longer interaction, it might also be helpful to invite Yolande to express more of her feelings about her husband and/or her own isolation by asking: 'I get the feeling you're quite worried about your husband and how he is, and perhaps anxious not to put pressure on him. What's he like, then, your Sam?', following this with other open and direct invitations to talk more about this important relationship. This would help the hospice team begin to develop a better understanding of Yolande's social circumstances and possible home care issues.

Sam's recent heart attack may both mean that Yolande has (temporarily?) lost an important source of social support, and also raise significant concerns for her about making him unwell if she returns home and he has to exert himself to care for her. It is possible that Yolande may feel guilty or worried at some level that her own illness was a contributory factor to her husband's recent heart attack. Expressing an interest in her relationship with her husband may be a useful way to open dialogue on these sensitive themes.

Case note 13

Sylvie Duvall was the mother of two children, Alain (9) and Dennis (4) by her long-term partner Didier. Sylvie was diagnosed with breast cancer, and had a mastectomy after radiotherapy. The oncologist was reassuring, explaining that she felt there was a good chance of 'full recovery' since the cancer had been caught 'at an early stage'. The oncologist suggested that after a few months they should meet again to discuss possible options for 'reconstructing' her breast for cosmetic reasons. In the meantime, Sylvie began long-term chemotherapy to help prevent recurrence.

Unfortunately, the surgery had required the excision of substantial lymph node tissue under one arm. As a result Sylvie developed problems with lymphodoema in her right arm. This produced chronic swelling in the arm as fluid accumulated, and the skin around her arm became coarser and pitted. Sylvie was very distressed to learn that the damage to the lymph nodes was irreversible. She was referred to a lymphodoema nurse for advice about bandaging and massage to help reduce the swelling, and over time formed a close relationship with the nurse, Hannah.

Although massage and bandaging helped reduce the swelling quite quickly, Hannah felt that Sylvie seemed lower in spirits with each visit. She commented on this, and Sylvie said: 'Yah, I do feel very down. I feel so ugly with all this, like an Egyptian mummy from the tomb. I haven't taken the kids swimming for ages. I really want to talk to Didier about it, but the more I try the more he seems to back off. I really feel like we're losing touch. His mother died of breast cancer, and I think if anything he's more scared than I am.'

Why we sometimes don't invite patients to share concerns

HCPs working in palliative care are sometimes reluctant to invite patients to share emotional or psychosocial problems. Some common reasons for this are that:

- they may feel it is not their role to do so;
- they may worry that they may be 'stirring up' the patient's distress in ways and making things worse;
- they may be concerned that they may not have the skills to deal with the response if they open a 'can of worms';
- they may be concerned that they have a big enough workload already without asking for more.

Clearly there is some interdependence between these factors. If the HCP works in a role seen by the organization as relating mainly to physical care and which requires a high case-load, the HCP may very genuinely find it problematic to encourage long conversations with patients about psychosocial concerns. They may also find it hard to gain easy access to training and support to develop good counselling skills.

Working from the relationship rather the role

In the case note presented, Hannah has already shown some very effective use of patient-centred counselling skills. First, by noticing a pattern developing over time, as Sylvie's mood changes. Second, by empathically 'reflecting' this back to invite a response at a psychological level. This gave Sylvie 'permission' or a cue that her feelings are a legitimate topic for discussion with a lymphodoema nurse. In doing this, Hannah has been led by her warm relationship with the patient rather than her technical role.

Active listening

Sylvie's disclosure is complex and rich, stating or hinting at many different kinds of loss and psychosocial issues. Good counselling skills include acknowledging and validating what the patient has communicated. That is, finding a way to let the patient know that they have been heard and understood at least to some degree, and that you are interested to try to understand more and better. In order to do this, the HCP must try to reflect on what the patient *means*, rather than simply parrot back the same words the patient has used in a display of listening and memory rather than understanding and empathy.

Listening attentively, Hannah would be able to hear concerns about:

- altered body image, which might relate both to Sylvie's self-image, and also to her feelings about how others may see her (Price 1995; Salter 1997);
- her relationship with her children and the impact of her illness and treatment on them;
- fear about the future (e.g. her reference to being scared and the mention of a tomb);
- her relationship with her partner Didier and the impact of her illness and treatment on him.

In particular, she is hinting at the development of a rather vicious circle between herself and Didier, perhaps fuelled by his own previous family experience of dealing with breast cancer. Sylvie may also be hinting at concerns about sexuality and physical intimacy, through her comments about feeling ugly and her remark that she and Didier are 'losing touch'. Perhaps this is not entirely metaphorical?

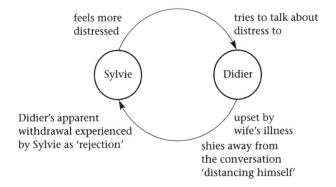

Figure 1 Vicious circle of approach/withdrawal

There have already been actual losses at a physical and psychological level (body parts, image of the self as an attractive, whole and healthy person). Sylvie is also troubled by potential or anticipatory losses: of good relationships with her children and partner, and perhaps of life itself. Hannah might also realize that some fears about the future might relate to future treatments. Some surgical reconstruction has been suggested, yet the conversation with Sylvie takes place precisely because of damaging side-effects from previous surgery, from the treatment received rather than the illness itself.

Hannah may feel overwhelmed

Given the intensity and complexity of the communication, there is a risk that Hannah might feel overwhelmed by the response, particularly if she knows two other patients are already sitting in reception, or if she is not particularly experienced or confident in handling such conversations. This might create some temptation to respond either by:

- rushing to refer the patient on to someone else seen as more 'expert' in therapeutic work ('Oh dear Sylvie, you've got a lot on your mind, haven't you? What I suggest is that you fix up a meeting with the counsellor here. She's a really nice person, with a lot more experience than me in talking through these things. Look, here's a leaflet about how to get in touch with her'), or
- keeping a low profile, to avoid encouraging further discussion ('Oh dear Sylvie, you've got a lot on your mind, haven't you? No wonder you're feeling down. Nearly finished with this arm now, hold still for just a minute more and then we'll be done today').

Hannah may try to be too helpful

Given the close relationship that has developed between Hannah and Sylvie through their one-to-one physical care sessions, there may also be some temptation to try to 'rescue' Hannah from her distress, by offering her rapid reassurance and comfort ('I think this is quite a common phase many people go through when they get lymphodoema – try not to worry too much. So long as you and Didier love each other, you'll find a way through'). Alternatively she may 'take on' Hannah's problems and try to develop solutions to them on the spot ('Oh, I can see what you mean about going swimming after the kind of surgery you've had. Have you spoken to Sue Fisher yet, the breast care nurse? She's got a lot of information about prosthetics, including special bathing costumes').

Empathic reflection of Sylvie's concerns, and permission/invitation to continue

More constructively, the next step for Hannah is to acknowledge Sylvie's distress and show that it is acceptable to talk further about such issues, if and when she would like to. Hannah might say: 'Sylvie, it does sound like you've got a lot on your mind – how this may be affecting Alain and Dennis, how things are between you and Didier, especially with his mother having died from breast cancer, and I suppose how you feel about yourself right now. You said that you're feeling really down – what's that like for you?' Another very valid approach might be to focus more specifically on the feeling cues offered: 'That does sound really hard Sylvie. You're feeling down, scared too, and by the sound of it pretty frustrated and worried.'

Seek to understand and connect with this patient here and now, before trying anything else

These responses do not preclude the subsequent offer of a referral to a counsellor, or the provision of information and/or referrals for other specialist expertise such as prosthetics services. Rather, the aim is to allow a space in which the meaning of Sylvie's communication can be allowed to unfold rather than being taken for granted – a space which takes the patient's feelings and wishes as the starting point. If we do not hear what these are to begin with, then any recommendations for advice or treatment are our own professional-led guesses and quick-fixes rather than patient-centred responses.

Exploring and clarifying concerns further

The development of the conversation should be led by Sylvie's subsequent responses. It may be that an empathic reflection or acknowledgement of Sylvie's distress is enough to allow Sylvie to develop her expression of concerns more fully. However, when a patient has offered such a range of cues about different concerns, it may also be helpful to ask the patient what concerns them most: 'I just wonder, with such a lot going on, what would you say is worrying you most of all at the moment?'

Containment through prioritizing and pacing

One way of helping patients to 'contain' or manage their distress when they face multiple problems is to support them to consider the problems one at a time, and to help the patient to think through each concern more fully. It may be helpful to encourage the patient to list the issues facing them on paper. Although this does not solve the problems, it may help bring some sense of order and manageability to the situation, and convey a sense that there are ways to begin to tackle a tangled multitude of problems stage by stage.

An alternative approach is to ask the patient to prioritize issues for discussion: 'I wonder if it might help to say a bit more about these problems. Where would be the best place to start?' This leaves the patient some choice between exploring the most dreaded issues, or approaching themes that may seem more manageable. Although this seems to offer the patient more control or choice in the conversation, there is a risk that the patient may not be able to share their most embarrassing/ frightening/least 'acceptable' concerns without some explicit permission or encouragement from their listener (Bor *et al.* 1998: 49).

A possible continuation

Suppose that Sylvie goes on to talk more about difficulties in her relationship with Didier:

Sylvie: 'Well, I just feel so depressed sometimes, especially when Didier and I have arguments or he won't talk to me. We used to be such a close couple.'

Hannah: 'It sounds like this illness pushes you apart at times. Could you say a bit more about how it's affected you as a couple?'

Sylvie: 'It's not just that we don't talk – I feel so ugly the whole time, and I get the feeling that he's really gone off me too.'

Hannah: 'What do you mean? Why do you think that?'

Sylvie: 'He's hardly touched me since I've had this operation, and this [points to arm]. I think he's really turned off by it, and I suppose I don't blame him. It feels like we're sleeping in different beds sometimes.'

Hannah: 'Do you think there might be any other reasons for what's happening between the two of you?'

Sylvie: 'I don't know really. I think he is very worried about the cancer and whether it might come back, and I think he's worried he might hurt me if we tried having sex. I've been quite sore where the scars are, and I've kind of dried up since I've been on these new drugs. We had quite a bad time when we tried, you know, tried a few weeks ago, it really hurt.'

Hannah: 'That's sounds really awful for both of you. I suppose I shouldn't be surprised that you and he are finding it tricky adjusting to things – I think a lot of couples have these kind of problems with sex and being intimate with illness and treatment like this. However, there is a lot that can be done to help. Sometimes even some quite simple changes like knowing what lubricant to use can make a big difference. Our information centre has got some good booklets and advice about resources that should help, and I know the Macmillan nurses here would be able to give you and Didier some more support and advice if you wanted. Would you like me to help you get in touch with them?'

Matters of timing and pacing

Note that at this point in the conversation it is entirely appropriate to offer some specific, limited advice about the problem, and to invite the patient to consider a referral for further more specialist support. From the exchange so far, Hannah has helped Sylvie to express and clarify her concerns and feel heard, has been led by the patient's priorities, and is now in a good position to offer the patient genuine reassurance and hope.

The role of the HCP as non-expert

With issues of sex and sexuality in palliative care, as with many other sensitive and potentially demanding themes, it is crucial that HCPs develop the confidence and skills to offer a contribution to patient care at an appropriate level for their position, training and relationship to the patient, rather than feeling constrained by an 'all or nothing' stark choice between being an expert and knowing nothing at all and feeling unable to help (van Ooijen 1996). In this example, Hannah has been following the widely used PLISSIT model of support for sexual needs in palliative care (Permission, Limited Information, Specialist Support, Intensive Therapy; MacElveen-Hoehn 1985).

The idea is that all professionals should be able to offer support at some level, with the most basic of these being Permission to explore and express needs and concerns about sexuality. A second step may be needed to provide 'Limited Information' (e.g. that a lubricant may be helpful, and that such difficulties are 'normal' and potentially treatable), then to offer links to 'Specialist Services' (e.g. information resources, Macmillan nursing), and to facilitate referral, if appropriate, to 'Intensive Therapies' (e.g. some couples may benefit from referral to a specialist psychosexual therapist if other measures do not alleviate the problem). Obviously Hannah is not a psychosexual therapist, but she can use her counselling skills to offer support through the other steps both directly and indirectly.

Other directions

Clearly, there are many other directions the conversation might take, depending on Sylvie's particular concerns. For example, she may reply that: 'I suppose I'm most worried about the children at the moment. They know something's wrong, but I don't think they know what. I don't really know what I should say to them.'

Bringing the conversation to a close

Later in the conversation, Hannah might ask: 'I don't think that we've talked about these things before. What's it been like for you sharing some of these feelings with me?'

Sylvie: 'Well, I'm sorry I've cried, I know you've got plenty to do and other people to see, but I am glad we've talked. I do feel so lonely sometimes and it's good to share that with someone. It just feels like Didier doesn't want to know.'

Hannah: 'I'm glad you think it's been useful – I think it is a part of my job, and I'd be happy to talk again like this when we next meet about your arm. If you find it does help to talk with someone, and you've got a lot of things to think through, I wonder if you might also want me to ask the counsellor to get in touch with you?'

Hannah validates Sylvie's use of her for discussing emotional and relationship issues, but also stays in role by framing this in the context of the lymphodoema work and offering a further referral to counselling.

Case note 14

Mr Crossover was a vicar who developed bowel cancer at the age of 61. Mr Crossover and his wife Ethel had been very well known and liked in the parish, and there was considerable sympathy for the couple when he announced his retirement through ill-health. He received radiotherapy, surgery to remove a section of diseased bowel and reroute the bowel to a stoma, and a course of chemotherapy. His treatment seemed to go very well, and he was told that he only needed to return for yearly check-ups with the oncology department. Ruth, the stoma care nurse, was pleased how well Mr Crossover learned to manage his stoma independently.

About four years after his operation Mr Crossover developed an infection and inflammation around the stoma site. Ruth resumed contact with him at the GP's request. She commented: 'It's a shame this has happened after you've had such a good run, but we'll be able to sort this out for you quite soon. I don't think it's anything to worry about too much.'

Mr Crossover nodded: 'Yes, that's what the doctor said. I was quite worried though, as I knew I was coming up to the five years and then I thought this might be the cancer coming back. It was very frightening. It's difficult to have much faith in the future any more. You just keep wondering what's round the corner.' Ruth asked politely how Mrs Crossover was doing. Mr Crossover replied: 'Oh, she's OK I think. I didn't worry her about this, as the whole messy business with the stoma upsets her, but that's not too much of a problem as we sleep in separate bedrooms now.'

What kinds of loss are potentially involved here?

There are several different kinds of loss which may be relevant for Ruth to consider here. One of the most obvious losses is that of normal bowel function following mutilating surgery, with possible issues of altered body image resulting from this. Mr Crossover suggests that this has been disturbing for his wife in some ways, but also hints that there has been a change in their relationship as a result: 'We sleep in separate bedrooms now.' It is not clear, however, whether he is implying that this has involved a significant or troubling loss of quality in their relationship, either in terms of sexual activity and/or physical intimacy, or whether his comment that they sleep separately now reflects a greater distance in their relationship more generally.

Professional-led versus patient-led agendas

Mr Crossover's remarks suggest that husband and wife have both found some degree of distancing and avoidance useful as coping strategies. This kind of hypothesis provides Ruth with some guide about areas for constructive discussion and exploration. It is important for professionals to focus on aspects which patients are indicating as their own priorities, rather than respond in ways which follow the professional's 'need to know'.

Ruth might ask: 'You say that this messy business with the stoma has upset your wife – in what ways?' as a way of acknowledging that issue and using an open question to invite further discussion. For example, are there specific concerns about physical intimacy (Burton and Watson 1998: 62–5), or does the stoma remind Mrs Crossover that she might be widowed? Have there been specific traumatic or embarrassing incidents involving spillage or bursting colostomy bags in public? Asking this kind of question might be a way of exploring whether the possible embarrassment or stigma of a cancer involving the bowel and faeces has led to other kinds of relationship losses, e.g. whether the couple have restricted their social life with other villagers because of concern about particular foods, accidents, etc.

Although this might be supportive in some ways, focusing on possible relationship changes between Mr Crossover and his wife runs a serious risk of following a professional-led agenda rather than responding to the patient's priorities. Mr Crossover had already volunteered powerful cues about his own feelings and concerns before Ruth asked about his wife. A focus on Mrs Crossover or the couple's relationship could be seen as a way in which the HCP is seeking to avoid or distract attention away from some more dreaded or difficult issues for the patient, or perhaps issues which Ruth would find more difficult to explore.

Loss of confidence in the future and in one's own body

Mr Crossover's words suggest strongly that he is troubled by other kinds of loss. It is notable how assertive he has been in politely acknowledging the reassurance that the GP and the stoma nurse have offered him, but then clearly stating some fears he has nonetheless. If Ruth listened carefully to the strong emotional cues that he offers (e.g. 'It was very frightening'), she should notice that Mr Crossover feels vulnerable and frightened about his future health. In a sense, his illness has made him lose the illusion of personal invulnerability that sustains many of us until we have a serious illness (Altschuler 1997: ch. 1). He has lost his image of himself as a healthy, fit person and may well have lost plans and confidence for the future that he may have harboured before illness when contemplating his retirement (Davy 1999).

This loss of confidence in the future, and loss of a self-image as a 'healthy' person, are major issues for many cancer patients, and yet can be easily overlooked by HCPs in their dealings with patients who appear to have made good 'recoveries' in physical terms. Particular crises of confidence may be triggered by new health events which may appear quite minor to an unempathic outsider, or may occur at times invested with particular social or cultural significance, for example, reaching 'normal' retirement age, or coming to a particular date after treatment which has been described by doctors, in the media or by others as having particular salience. Many patients invest a great deal of significance in reaching 'five years' without a recurrence, since this is a period often cited in morbidity and mortality statistics.

Loss of faith

In addition to a loss of confidence in the future or in the self as a healthy person, it is also possible that Mr Crossover is trying to find a way of speaking about a spiritual concern, a loss of faith (Anon. 1991). His words could be heard simply as an expression of anxiety about the future, but it is also possible that he is saying something about losing a whole set of sustaining beliefs about the world and his place in it (Wright *et al.* 1996). After a lifetime of service to God, how does Mr Crossover make sense of his own illness? Has his illness shaken his faith in God entirely, or might Mr Crossover still believe but doubt his own place in the here-after? When he speaks of worrying about 'what is round the corner', might he be referring to heaven, hell or oblivion (Kearney 1996)?

Being led by the patient

The cues Mr Crossover has offered about these themes seem much stronger than those about any relationship concerns. It is impor-tant to note that he has volunteered these unprompted. More accurately, he has asserted these concerns in the face of attempted reassurance that he should not worry. Responding to these key concerns, Ruth might say something like: 'Hmm, I suppose it's all too easy for other people like me to try to be reassuring and positive, but I guess in your shoes it feels very different. I don't think I'd appreciated how much you were thinking about this five-year business, and how much you are frightened and worry-ing about the future. Would you like to say some more about that?', or perhaps more briefly but with the same intent: 'I'm sorry, I hadn't appreciated how worried you are. What do you think might be round the corner?'

Both offer a congruent acknowledgement that she and others may have inappropriately reassured Mr Crossover, reflect back that she hears the depth of his concern, and give permis-sion for him to proceed if he wishes. It is very unlikely that in so doing Ruth will be 'stirring up' new concerns for Mr Crossover. He has suggested clearly that he already finds himself troubled by some issues, but has been unable to share these with his wife or GP.

Remaining curious about the patient's own resources

After inviting Mr Crossover to voice his concerns more fully, Ruth may then ask: 'How do you go about trying to manage these fears?', as a way of assessing future support needs, and as an invitation to Mr Crossover to reflect on his internal and social resources. Encouraging patients to reflect on what does work for them may be very empowering in its own right, both in terms of helping patients take credit for their own actions, and also because it is easier for patients to 'do more of what works' if they are helped to name and notice it (George *et al.* 1990).

Mr Crossover: 'Well, I suppose the last time I felt like this I was lucky, because my old friend Father Brian from Ullander was visiting. He was a marvellous prop for my faith, very down to earth but inspirational too.'

Ruth: 'Do you think it might be useful to get in touch with him now, or someone like him?'

Mr Crossover: 'Well, I don't like to bother people too much, but I suppose he wouldn't mind. I've got his e-mail address – perhaps I should get in touch, if only to wish him the season's greetings.'

Noticing what doesn't work

Conversely, supporting patients to notice ineffective strategies may be a way of enabling them to abandon these and try something different in a more empowering way than offering expert advice about what patients should and shouldn't do. For example:

Mr Crossover: 'Well, I've tried prayer, but frankly I just get more worked up – the words won't come any more, and I'm not sure my heart's really in it.'

Ruth: 'Do you think it will be useful to keep trying, or would it be better to take a break for a while?'

Mr Crossover: 'No, I don't think I should take a break as you put it. Prayer is very important to me, but I think God listens to different kinds of prayers, and maybe it's time for me to offer prayers in a different way.'

Ruth: 'Such as?' (and so on)

Supporting spiritual reflection rather than advising

By asking such questions, motivated by a genuine curiosity rather than a desire to guide Mr Crossover to a predetermined answer, Ruth can help Mr Crossover to consider these highly charged spiritual issues, without feeling that she has to be an expert on religious faith or spiritual guidance. If it is clear that Mr Crossover is wrestling with matters of religious faith, it may be appropriate to ask: 'I suppose other vicars will have doubts like these from time to time. What advice would you give a colleague in a similar position?'

Such an invitation to consider problems from a different perspective is another empowering way to support patients to share and consider their needs. While acknowledging the concern, the HCP helps the patient to take one step back to get a different view.

Reconnecting Mr Crossover's concerns to relationship issues

Later in the conversation, Ruth might ask questions such as: 'Are there other people that you have been able to discuss these concerns with?' and: 'Do you think it's helpful to talk with someone about these fears?', as ways to explore what further support Mr Crossover might need. Similarly, questions such as: 'Are there any ways in which it might be helpful for your wife if you did share some of these concerns with her?' or even: 'You said you were worried this might be cancer coming back. If that did happen, how do you think that might affect Mrs Crossover?' could offer a way to explore some of the relationship issues and possible future challenges for the couple.

Main learning points

- Patients, family and staff in palliative care face many different kinds of loss, both current and anticipated. HCPs need to develop their awareness of the range of possible losses.

- Losses may include changes in relationships, beliefs or self-images, in addition to more physical losses.
- The significance of any particular kind of loss may vary hugely between individuals. HCPs must avoid filtering patients' experiences through their own values and beliefs.
- HCPs must be careful not to block discussions which involve losses they find particularly distressing to contemplate.
- Where patients seem overwhelmed by multiple losses, it may be important to help them list and rank these losses, and help pace the review of these.
- Patients may choose to disclose and discuss sensitive issues of loss with any staff member, often depending more on the warmth and trust they feel in the relationship rather than the professional's official role.
- Sometimes intimate physical care facilitates relationships of trust in which patients may disclose significant vulnerabilities.
- Every HCP needs good counselling skills so that we can be patient-led. This does not imply that all HCPs should be 'experts' in counselling. As with the PLISSIT model of supporting sexual concerns, all HCPs should be able to offer constructive and containing responses *and* know how to refer on for specialist advice if needed.
- Exploration of previous changes or losses in life may raise the person's awareness of their coping patterns.
- Listening to the language patients use in communicating their concerns can offer clues as to the meaning of their anxieties.

Chapter 5

Symptom management

Introduction

Palliative care patients and their carers may be affected by a very wide range of symptoms. These are not simply a function of the particular disease (and treatments) involved. We need to consider what support systems and coping strategies are available, and the impact of symptoms on the lives of patients and their loved ones. In particular, we must strive to understand the *meanings* that patients attribute to their symptoms.

Palliative care aims to alleviate symptoms as far as possible. However, we must be careful not to be drawn into treating symptoms and problems, rather than treating whole *people* who are affected by symptoms.

The two examples in this chapter show how symptoms may carry several meanings simultaneously, and call for responses from HCPs that take into account both physical processes and psychosocial issues.

Case note 15

Mrs Easterman was a 70-year-old woman with a fungating tumour to one side of her neck. She had received a variety of treatments over the two years since her diagnosis, which had kept its growth in check for a while. However, it was clear that the tumour could not actually be removed completely. Her doctors believed that the tumour would eventually grow to block Mrs Easterman's windpipe totally, or more probably until it infiltrated the major blood vessels of her neck.

Mrs Easterman lived at home by herself, and had remained mobile, active and self-caring in spite of her disease. Her husband had died some ten years previously, but Mrs Easterman's son and daughter lived locally and visited from time to time. Mrs Easterman was well known in the local community as a stalwart of her church, and received many other visitors. She was known to the local hospice through the Macmillan nurse team, but generally received most of her palliative care through her GP's practice and Mavis, the district nurse who visited daily to change the dressings on her neck.

Generally Mrs Easterman presented as a lively and articulate woman with a keen sense of humour, laced with a rather acid wit. Mavis had made many visits to Mrs Easterman's home, and had often heard her talking about her deceased husband, her family, and about her working life as a book-binder. However, Mrs Easterman seldom talked about her illness and the future, even when her dressing was being changed, when she swapped tales about TV soap stars with Mavis.

One day while Mavis was changing the dressing Mrs Easterman winced and pulled away. Mavis apologized. Mrs Easterman said: 'It's looking bigger today, isn't it? I could feel it pulsing last night, and I couldn't sleep a wink. I try not to think about what's going to happen, but sometimes I just get so frightened.'

Focus on the meaning of symptoms

In using counselling skills to help patients manage symptoms, it is crucial that we think in terms of the significance and meaning of a symptom for a patient, not just the apparent 'objective', physical facts (Barry 1996). Although Mrs Easterman is able to 'function' well day to day and does not at present suffer major pain or physical disability from the tumour, it is evident that even quite small changes in the tumour may carry great significance in terms of prompting Mrs Easterman to think about an unpleasant future.

In this situation, a poor response would be to ignore the risk Mrs Easterman has taken in admitting her fear. Mrs Easterman has already told us that this is not a new concern, but rather one that has been on her mind for a while even though she usually tries to push it away. Mavis might be tempted to say: 'I'm sorry you had a bad night. I wonder what we can do today to help you take your mind off things? There's going to be a concert at the hospice tomorrow – would you like to go to that?', and/or perhaps offer reassurance and an offer of 'making things better': 'I am sorry I was a bit clumsy then, I didn't mean to hurt you. Your neck doesn't really look much different to me. Would you like me to ask the doctor about some sleeping pills for tonight, just in case?'

Both of these responses are well intentioned, and it may indeed be helpful to offer Mrs Easterman distraction activities and night-time medication at some point. However, to do so immediately blocks further communication at an emotional or psychological level about a very frightening symptom (Faulkner and Maguire 1994: ch. 2). Mrs Easterman is clearly communicating that her usual tactic of self-distraction and avoidance is not sufficient for her at this point.

Whose 'role' is it to respond?

Mavis might believe that psychological support is more the role of the Macmillan team, and ask: 'Have you talked about that with your Macmillan nurse before?' Exploring the patient's use of other resources in the caring network is quite appropriate if used as a complement to the HCP's own response, but problematic if used to block further discussion or to 'pass the buck' (Mrs Easterman: 'No, not really.' Mavis: 'When is she next due to visit you? If I were you, I'd let her know you're worried about it then, and

see what she has to say. They're just the right people for that sort
of thing.')

Giving the patient honest feedback about their condition

Mrs Easterman seems to be asking for some feedback from the
HCP about the progression of the tumour. Failing to answer the
question may collude with the fear that the tumour itself is something too terrible to discuss. In order to deliver patient-centred
care, we must have faith in the patient and accept that, when we
are asked a direct question, patients want us to deal openly and
honestly with it.

   If the tumour seems no different in size to Mavis, she might
reply: 'Well, in all honesty I haven't noticed the tumour looking
any bigger recently, but I appreciate you're thinking about
how it might be growing within you, and how it will get bigger
over time. I think I can see how frightening it is to think about
that at times. What do you imagine might happen, and what
worries you most about that?' If the tumour does appear larger,
a simple acknowledgement of this might be a powerful and
genuine enough response: 'Yes, I think it is looking bigger,'
although this could constructively be linked with an invitation
to discuss: 'What is your greatest fear about what might happen?'
A major aim here is simply to empower the patient to articulate
her fears, at a pace that is sensitive to Mrs Easterman's readiness
to do this.

A dilemma in asking about dreaded issues

The HCP might choose to ask the same questions but with a
slightly gentler pace by first asking: 'Tell me, what were you thinking about last night?', before inviting Mrs Easterman to say what
is most frightening about this. When we slow down the approach
to asking about most dreaded issues, it is important to be mindful
whether this is being done for the patient's sake, or whether it
may reflect our own unease or distress at what we might hear. If
the HCP asks about the patient's fears in a very roundabout way,

this may communicate to the patient that the HCP has difficulty engaging with the issues, and might inadvertently lead the patient to protect the HCP by hiding or minimizing some of their fears (Bor *et al.* 1998: ch. 6).

Use open rather than closed or leading questions

The HCP needs to be able to listen attentively and with genuine curiosity to the answers that Mrs Easterman may give. If the HCP makes the mistake of assuming that Mrs Easterman is most frightened of dying, or for example most frightened of choking to death, this may hinder the HCP's ability to hear and respond to the patient. For this reason, it is better to ask open questions that do not invite or presume a particular response (Faulkner and Maguire 1994: ch. 4), rather than closed or leading questions ('I can see why you might be frightened – with a tumour like this, are you worried about choking to death?').

By way of illustration, imagine two quite different fears that Mrs Easterman might hold. She might reply: 'Well, the thing that keeps me awake at night is worrying about how I will, well, how I will actually, die, when the time comes . . . I just can't help thinking that I'm going to drown in my own blood, just like a horror movie. I'm sorry, that's such an awful thing to say, but I can't help thinking about it and I'm so scared.'

Equally, however, she might reveal other concerns which would otherwise be unguessable to the HCP: 'Well, I'm not worried about dying, not really, I've had a long time to think about that – but I just don't know whether I'll see Arthur again afterwards. He was such a good man and I'm sure he's in heaven, but I've done some very bad things in my life, things he never knew about. I'm scared I might be going to the other place.'

The former concern might be responded to through an open discussion about how the tumour might progress, and what might happen at the time of her death. However, the latter concern would strongly suggest the value of seeking spiritual guidance for Mrs Easterman through her church, a palliative care team chaplain, or possibly a counsellor.

Closing the conversation

In closing the conversation with Mrs Easterman, it may be helpful to say something like: 'I'm glad that we were able to talk about this a bit today, it's certainly helped me appreciate how it feels for you at the moment. I appreciate that you do like to talk about other things as well, but I wanted to let you know I'd be very happy to talk about this again if you like.' This contains a respectful acknowledgement of Mrs Easterman's usual coping strategy, while offering a bridge to other future conversations about the patient's fears. Mavis might also ask: 'Would it be useful to let anyone else know you've been thinking like this?' This encourages Mrs Easterman to consider what support she could seek from other HCPs or family and friends. It may also help her reflect whether there are important conversations to be had with other family members if she is becoming more able to admit that her time may be quite limited.

Case note 16

Mr Jones is a 54-year-old man with cancer of the pancreas diagnosed six months previously. He has already been admitted to the hospice twice for assessment and treatment of significant pain. Both times he returned home to his wife with his pain apparently well under control through a careful combination of medication and the use of a TENS machine, but each time after a few days his wife telephoned the hospice team reporting that Mr Jones was 'in terrible pain' and begging for him to be re-admitted.

Mr Jones is admitted for a third time. While the doctor is clerking him in, Asha the nurse is talking with Mrs Jones in a side-room. Mrs Jones is in floods of tears, and seems barely able to talk, gulping for air between sobs. Asha sits with her quietly until the tears subside enough for Mrs Jones to talk more freely, and says: 'Mrs Jones, I'm really sorry that things seem to have got so bad again at home. We'll do everything we can to help. Can you tell me what's been happening?' Mrs Jones says: 'I just can't bear seeing him like this. He used to be such a fit man, so well built, and now look at him, he hardly weighs anything and he's in such pain all the time. You wouldn't treat a dog like this, he's got no quality of life, we're just waiting for the end. It's criminal. There must be a way, surely, that the doctor can do something to help him die? He's too proud to ask, he wouldn't want to be difficult, but he's in such pain all the time and I just wish we could end it. You say you'll do everything you can, well help him properly this time then, don't just give him a pill and send him home again.'

Euthanasia

Mrs Jones raises a common but emotive issue in palliative care, that of euthanasia. In the current British legal context, it is against the law for anyone, including healthcare professionals (HCPs), actively to assist someone else to die where this is the main aim of the intervention. At the risk of oversimplifying a complex legal position, it is not illegal to administer treatments to a patient which may have the side-effect of shortening life, if the principal aim of the treatment is not to kill but rather to alleviate a symptom. Thus it is legal to administer high doses of morphine to a patient in significant pain, even where this carries some risk of depressing respiratory function, but it is not legal to administer a drug such as morphine in order to kill a patient even if this is what they request (NCHSPCS 1993 and 1997 offer further consideration of such ethical issues).

Many palliative care professionals are profoundly opposed to euthanasia, viewing it as a measure which may be sought in desperation when effective palliative care is unavailable. Other workers may oppose euthanasia but support the legalization of assisted suicide as a valid way to offer patients greater autonomy over the manner of their death complementary to care enhancing quality of life (see Dickenson and Johnson 1993: chs 29–32).

The issue of euthanasia may also be especially highly charged for both professionals and patients/carers because of religious and cultural beliefs in addition to legal codes. Experienced palliative care workers may develop quite ambivalent yet unacknowledged feelings about euthanasia as they repeatedly encounter patients who experience distressing and unpleasant deaths despite good palliative care support, and their early idealistic commitment to the possibilities of palliative care is repeatedly tested against a capricious reality.

A forbidden topic

Because euthanasia is such a loaded issue, some palliative care workers are very reluctant to discuss it. This can be unhelpfully reflected in their communications with patients and carers. Asha might say: 'Mrs Jones, you know that's illegal and that's not something we should be discussing,' or: 'Mrs Jones, we don't support the idea of euthanasia, which is illegal anyway. What we should be thinking about is how to help Mr Jones feel as comfortable as possible.'

These defensive responses represent an attempt by the professional to maintain their own perceived integrity, but at the expense of the patient and carer. Mrs Jones may well feel ignored and patronized, and is unlikely to feel reassured that the palliative care team will take her concerns seriously. These insensitive responses may exacerbate guilt that Mrs Jones might already be feeling for wishing that her husband would die, and might well anger her further at a time when she is faced with major loss and has already had to deal with two abortive attempts to discharge her husband home to her care.

Collusion

If Asha is actually sympathetic to the idea of euthanasia, another kind of error would be to offer collusive support against the rest of the palliative care team. For example: 'I'm really sorry, Mrs Jones, if I could help I would. I think everyone has a right to end things if they want, but I'm not in charge here.' This will further undermine Mrs Jones' confidence in the quality of care that can be provided. While this may seem a rather obvious error, a close relationship with a patient over time and a genuine perception that the patient is suffering may tempt HCPs into such responses as an angry reflection of their own feelings of impotence.

Using empathy rather than sympathy

Instead of colluding with or opposing Mrs Jones' plea for euthanasia, Asha needs to respond by valuing and accepting Mrs Jones' feelings and concerns. Importantly, accepting someone's concerns need not imply agreeing with the solutions that they propose. This reflects an important distinction between an empathic understanding (which involves an attempt to understand how it might feel to be in someone else's shoes), as against sympathy (which involves the worker developing the same feelings or understanding of the situation as another person). Empathy is an attempt to understand as if one was the other, while still retaining a separate perspective and an awareness of this, while sympathy implies that one actually begins to feel and agree with the other (Tschudin 1987: ch. 4).

Respond at the level of feelings

In seeking to understand how it might feel to be in Mrs Jones' shoes at this point, Asha might recognize that she may be angry (both because her husband is dying, and because health services appear to be letting them down), sad and lonely at the losses facing her, and also frightened (in anticipation of her bereavement, on behalf of her husband and his pain, and perhaps in fear at the weight of responsibility that she has been asked to bear in caring for her husband each time he has been sent home). A response at this level of feeling reflects a good use of counselling skills, in contrast with a response at a 'factual' level arguing the rights and wrongs of euthanasia.

For example, Asha might say: 'I appreciate that it's really distressing seeing your husband this ill. I get the feeling that you may be really quite angry and perhaps frightened at what's been happening, and you're very concerned about what'll happen next.' The intention here is simply to try to acknowledge the depth and type of feeling, rather than offer solutions. It is possible that Mrs Jones may show more anger: 'Well of course I'm bloody angry – I'm furious that you keep sending him home when he's so ill, it's unbelievable.' While this would be uncomfortable for Asha, it would provide Mrs Jones a space in which she can express her anger at what is happening. This may also help the palliative care team understand the home care situation better.

When this intensity of feeling is present, it is usually a mistake to try to avoid it or pretend it is not there. Equally, it would then be a mistake to retaliate by criticizing Mrs Jones for showing these feelings. Asha's response has not caused Mrs Jones to become angry. Rather, in naming anger as one of the emotions present, some permission has been given to show and explore feelings that are already present (Stedeford 1994: ch. 10).

A fear that pain always worsens up until death

Mrs Jones might respond instead: 'Yes, I'm terrified. I've never had to deal with anything like this before, and I get so frightened when he's in pain, I just don't know what to do.'

Asha: 'What worries you most about that?'
Mrs Jones: 'Well, I know that he's going to be in more pain as the illness goes on, so I'm really worried what it'll be like when he's dying. I won't be able to cope with him at home then.'
Asha: 'I see. I know that a lot of people assume that pain does get worse as illness progresses, but it may be important for you to know that isn't necessarily so. I can see why you'd be very worried about having him at home if you think that'd mean him dying in a lot of pain. I think I'd better arrange for you to have some time to talk more with the doctor and with our home care team, so we can let you know about the different kinds of support we can offer when someone is dying at home, or when they die here in the hospice.'

Clearly this does not resolve the concerns Mrs Jones has expressed. However, the exchange does offer some immediate acknowledgement of her fears. Asha also conveys that these will be taken seriously and that Mrs Jones will be given more information and opportunities to ask questions. It also opens the way for discussion of where Mr Jones should be cared for until his death. Asha is not drawn into offering guarantees that she is not empowered to make (e.g. that Mr Jones will not be discharged again), but neither does she dismiss Mrs Jones' very understandable concerns about her husband's future care needs. Asha cannot honestly promise Mrs Jones that her husband's pain will not intensify, but she does offer genuine feedback that this is a common fear which may not materialize, and can be explored further with members of the palliative care team.

Who 'owns' the symptom?

It is important that Asha should not feel paralysed by a responsibility for 'curing' Mr Jones' symptoms or be defensive about the care that has been provided. In this encounter, her patient is effectively Mrs Jones. Asha's role is to help Mrs Jones express and clarify her distress and feel that this will be taken seriously by the whole team. One could conceptualize this as a case in which the palliative care team has been trying hard to focus on the symptoms of the cancer patient, but may not have given enough attention to Mrs Jones' experience of these symptoms, or indeed to the emotional 'symptoms' that Mrs Jones shows. These deserve good care every bit as much as Mr Jones' symptoms.

Disease affects the patient, but illness is a shared experience

In delivering holistic care that respects people's family and social context, we must appreciate that although disease is a physical process affecting the patient, illness is a shared experience which may affect everyone in the caring network (Davy 1999: 29). In some respects it is misleading to speak of Mr Jones' pain. Rather, Mr Jones' pancreatic disease has led to pain symptoms affecting both Mr and Mrs Jones, although in different ways. Mrs Jones' pain is psychological and emotional rather than a matter of sensory nerve firing, but it is clearly hard to bear.

Asha might go on to ask: 'Could you tell me some more about what it's been like at home when he's in pain – how does he show that . . . and what happens then . . . and how does that affect you?', to help Mrs Jones tell her side of the story, while also inviting a conversation which could shed some light on how Mr Jones' pain is managed at home.

Total pain

The ideas above reflect a view of pain as something influenced and experienced as a result of the interaction between a range of factors, some biological (e.g. tissue invasion and nerve involvement, physiological responses to analgesia), some psychological (e.g. what a person thinks it means that they have pain, or what beliefs they have about how this may change or be treated over time), and some social (e.g. whether a patient is being cared for in surroundings that match their preferences and culture, how other people respond to the patient's experience of pain). Together, these constitute 'clinical pain' or 'total pain' (Woodruff 1997: ch. 4).

Although this understanding of pain offers a richer way of understanding pain management and more ways of intervening, it also carries with it a risk of 'over-psychologizing' pain – being too ready to ascribe pain management problems to social and emotional circumstances rather than disease pathology.

It is tempting to blame others when things are going wrong

It is quite possible that a palliative care team under pressure might begin to attribute problems in pain management to Mrs Jones. The team may wonder whether she 'over-reacts' and magnifies minor expressions of pain by Mr Jones, and speculate whether his pain is aggravated by Mrs Jones' anxiety and manner with him. There is an understandable but unhelpful temptation to blame other people when something is going wrong. In this instance, Mr Jones' distress is leading Mrs Jones to blame the palliative care team, and it would be easy to imagine the care team beginning to blame Mrs Jones ('He'd be fine at home if only she didn't make such a fuss. We get him nicely settled here, and then when he goes home she gets so worked up it's no wonder he's getting stressed').

In talking with Mrs Jones, Asha must be careful to monitor her own beliefs about the situation and avoid questioning her in ways which will imply that she is at fault. Asha may also have a role to play in subsequent team discussions to help represent Mrs Jones' experience fairly and fully rather than reporting it critically.

Main learning points

- The impact of a symptom on a patient is not simply related to its current physical aspects. It is necessary to understand what *meaning* the patient attributes to the symptom, and how they believe the symptom may develop.
- Although disease refers to physical processes in a patients, illness affects all those in the social network. It can be helpful to consider what 'symptoms' relatives may have which require support.
- HCPs who have built a relationship of trust with their patients through close physical care may be well placed to support patients by attending to the meanings they attribute to their symptoms.
- Open questions help patients to express their concerns at their own pace. In contrast, closed or leading questions tend to reinforce the HCP's own prior assumptions or professional-led agenda.
- Pain is influenced by a range of biological, psychological and social factors. HCPs must attend to the interaction of these factors in order to understand the patient's 'total pain', maximizing their opportunities for supportive interventions.
- Euthanasia and the related issue of assisted suicide are common and emotive themes in palliative care, but may be hard to discuss openly for all concerned. If HCPs are reluctant to talk about these themes, this will inhibit patients and family

members from expressing serious concerns and may create further anxieties about symptom management and the manner of death.

- It is tempting to blame others when something is going wrong (or for carers to blame themselves if their loved one is suffering). HCPs must monitor their reactions to distressing situations and avoid implying that others are at fault. Blame invites blame in return.

Chapter **6**

Anger

Introduction

Many people can readily understand how frightened people may become when facing life-threatening illness. However, it seems harder for healthcare professionals (HCPs) to acknowledge the depths of anger that arise, particularly when this is directed towards the HCP, or when it is the HCP who feels anger towards the patient.

Anger can be a powerful assault on the self-images that sustain us in such emotionally demanding work. We like to believe that we care for our patients, and that patients appreciate the help we give them. However, to deny ourselves and patients the right to be angry in highly distressing circumstances is both naïve and disrespectful (Stedeford 1994: ch. 10).

This chapter uses three examples to examine how we as HCPs may try to make sense of anger and work with this emotion therapeutically rather than avoid it, retaliate or become defensive.

Case note 17

Mr Arbogast was a 77-year-old man with cancer of the prostate and associated metastases in his bones. He lived alone in a second-floor flat. He was admitted to the hospice for assessment and management of pain problems. Initially he responded well to changed medication and was looking forward to going home within days. However, while in the hospice, Mr Arbogast developed loss of sensation and power in his legs due to spinal cord compression. Palliative radiotherapy was rapidly arranged. Mr Arbogast regained better sensation and a little strength in his legs, but remained bedbound. He told Maria the occupational therapist that he was frightened he would fall.

Mr Arbogast's 'planned short admission' turned into a stay of many weeks as Maria and the team tried unsuccessfully to encourage Mr Arbogast to exercise and remobilize. It seemed unlikely that Mr Arbogast would be able to return to his own home unless he could make progress in this way. Mr Arbogast was adamant that he did not want to seek other accommodation and angrily refused to discuss care options with the social worker on several occasions. He began to complain of worsening pain problems, pressing the bedside buzzer with increasing frequency to complain that he needed different or more medication to control this. He became a very unpopular patient and many staff began to avoid passing by his bed unless summoned by the buzzer. Other patients nearby began to complain about him.

Maria came to dislike Mr Arbogast and dreaded the time she had to spend with him on rehabilitation exercises when he seemed sullen and uncooperative. One day when he answered her only with grunts, she lost her temper and said: 'Oh Mr Arbogast, for goodness sake make an effort, please. What is the point of my coming if you won't at least try?' He glared at her fiercely and replied: 'Fine, don't bother. Make yourself scarce like the rest of them do all the time. Bugger off and leave me to die in peace.'

Cycles of frustration and disappointment

It is easy for a sense of frustration or disappointment to creep into the health care team when patients experience setbacks, and professional efforts seem in vain. If our sense of job satisfaction comes from helping patients to feel better and maintain independence, a patient who is in pain, ungrateful, and lacking hope may unsettle us. In these circumstances, professional frustration can quickly translate into anger against the patient. The case note above is not simply about an angry patient. There is an escalating spiral of anger and bad feeling between the patient and the team. At each stage, the hostility and disappointment of one party may then ratchet up the distress of the other, and so on, in a 'vicious circle'.

Most of us are familiar with this pattern from some aspects of our private lives or family experience. In the palliative care environment, tempers may become especially heated because so much is at stake.

Anger may provoke fight or flight

A response such as: 'I'm sorry to have disturbed you Mr Arbogast, I'll come back later and see how you're feeling then' may appear to provide Maria with a polite exit from the scene, but fails to offer support and understanding to the patient and does nothing to interrupt the pattern that is developing between the patient and his carers. It also implies that the difficulties lie with Mr Arbogast's feelings alone. Worse, Maria might be drawn to 'retaliate' and escalate the conflict further by defending herself and the team: 'Mr Arbogast, I really don't think that's fair of you. I appreciate you're ill and in a difficult position, but we are doing our best and I'm sure that no-one is trying to avoid you. We're all professionals here.' The former represents flight and the latter fight in the well-known tendency for hostile situations to provoke people to prepare for 'fight or flight'. We might notice in passing that although flight is an option for the HCPs, this is not an option for in-patients except in a limited form through social withdrawal.

Self-reflexivity and compassion

One of the most important counselling skills is self-reflexivity. This means an ability to reflect on and make sense of one's own emotions and responses to situations, and a willingness to notice the effects of one's own contribution. In this situation, it is important that Maria can admit to herself that she is becoming angry and is starting to 'take this out' on the patient. This capacity can be supported by another important counselling skill, that of remaining non-judgemental about things which we may not like or support. Although it is a commonplace to argue that HCPs should try to be non-judgemental about patients and families, we must extend this courtesy to ourselves as well. If we can remain compassionate and non-judgemental about our own apparent failings, it is easier to notice them and either correct them or put them to good use.

Acknowledging the distress

Even if Maria feels too distressed or angry to stay with the situation, she might at least say: 'I'm really sorry that you're angry and upset at the moment Mr Arbogast. I appreciate that you are in a very difficult position here, and I think I'm not helping by getting cross like this myself. I'd like to come back later today when I've managed to get myself in a better frame of mind, and really try to get a better understanding of how you are and how we can improve our care for you. May I do that?' This acknowledges the feelings on both sides, and Maria's responsibility to work with the patient rather than against them, and holds out the clear message that Maria will persevere with the relationship in a way that is not contingent on Mr Arbogast being 'better behaved'. Even if Maria feels unable to stay with Mr Arbogast, it is important not to end the conversation in a way that blames him.

Persevering

More positively, Maria might say: 'I'm sorry that you're angry Mr Arbogast, and I think I've not been helping by getting cross like this myself. I apologize for that. If you really do want me to go away now I will do that and come back to talk to you later, but I'd rather stay with you so I can work out better ways for us to support you.' While this leaves Mr Arbogast the choice of sending her away, it assertively suggests that there is possibility and value to persisting, and conveys a message that Maria is not afraid to deal with the difficult emotions that are present. This response begins to interrupt the vicious circle of escalating tempers, without pretending that it has not happened; hence it is congruent as well as compassionate.

Externalizing

It might also be helpful to offer a comment such as: 'I think an illness like this can be very frustrating for everyone to deal with, and if we're not careful we end up getting upset with each other rather than the illness.' This suggests a more constructive way of understanding the situation than blaming each other, by naming the illness rather than Mr Arbogast as the problem. Separating the problem from the person in this way is known as 'externalizing' (White 1989) and may open the way to ask more questions about ways in which 'the illness has been affecting your life . . .' and how 'you and I can help you stop the illness running the show'.

One possible drawback to 'blaming the illness' rather than the patient in a case like this is that it may seem to invalidate Mr Arbogast's perception that the HCPs are avoiding him. This concern deserves an immediate response if Mr Arbogast is willing to continue the conversation, and a change in the way the team works with him. Maria might ask: 'You said that people seem to be making themselves scarce – what did you mean by that . . . how do you feel when that happens . . . why do you think that happens?'

This exploration also needs to be linked with action which could include (a) Maria contributing to team meetings to help her colleagues appreciate the impact of their behaviour on Mr Arbogast and consider ways to approach the situation differently, (b) accepting and exploring in more depth what Mr Arbogast's concerns are, and (c) Maria and/or other team members making a point of interrupting the cyclical pattern of angry/frightened demand by spending time alongside Mr Arbogast which is not just in response to his buzzer-pressing.

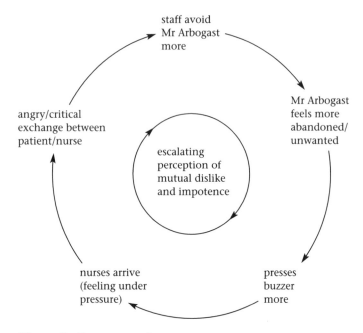

Figure 2   Buzzer-pressing

'Resistance' as feedback about helper inflexibility or ignorance

It is useful to understand apparent 'resistance' (or 'problem behaviours') on the part of patients as a way in which patients try to help us by communicating that we have not yet understood their concerns, or have not yet found the right way to help them (de Shazer 1984). From this perspective, 'resistance' does not call for greater force by the professional to overcome this, but rather calls for a renewed curiosity, exploration and empathy.

It is not difficult to imagine some reasons why Mr Arbogast might be angry in the situation described. He is in pain, feels ignored or rejected, may well feel that the health system has let him down, may be angry at his own weakness or failing body, and is probably very frightened, which can often be shown as anger when flight is not possible.

Helping him and the team untangle and separate these

issues and feelings may lead to more possibilities for intervention than interpreting Mr Arbogast simply as a 'difficult' patient. Note in particular that if Mr Arbogast does not feel that the team has taken all of his concerns seriously, it would be very understandable for him to lack confidence in the services and fear his own capacity to cope if discharged home.

Case note 18

Errol was a 48-year-old marketing executive who lived with his youngest daughter Bethany (15). His ex-wife had left him three years earlier and left the country. Bethany's older sister and brother were away at university in the south. Last year Errol was diagnosed with a slow-growing, inoperable brain tumour. He suffered from frequent severe headaches, nausea and dizziness. Bright light and movement around him seemed to exacerbate these problems, and Errol stayed indoors much of the time and had retired because of ill-health.

Marsha the Macmillan nurse visited occasionally to monitor the situation and to help the GP and Errol review medication needs. Errol seemed to appreciate this support very much. Marsha hardly ever saw Bethany, but often heard her elsewhere in the house, slamming doors loudly and playing raucous music at high volume.

Towards the end of one particularly noisy visit, Marsha commented good-naturedly to Errol: 'Wow, she is loud isn't she? I'm amazed you manage to get any rest with all this racket. I've got younger ones at home and they're bad enough, I dread the day they turn teenage and discover grunge or whatever this is!' Errol looked at her sadly and said: 'She wasn't like this before I became ill. Never you worry though, it's not so bad, she'll be quieter once you've gone. She's really good to me, really helpful, although it does bother me that she keeps skipping school so much.'

Rather guiltily, Marsha wondered if she should make more effort to meet and talk with Bethany, and with Errol's permission she knocked on Bethany's bedroom door before

> she left. When the daughter appeared, Marsha smiled pleasantly, and said: 'Hi Bethany, I was just wondering if I could talk with you for a few minutes? I'd like to see how you are and if there's anything we can do for you with your father being ill and all.' Bethany muttered: 'We're doing just fine without you, I wish you'd just go away and leave us alone,' and shut the door. The music volume surged.

Don't escalate

As with the previous example, a brief pause for reflection is required, rather than a continuation or escalation of this sequence. An unhelpful response at this point would be to knock more loudly on Bethany's door, and seek to continue the conversation; in effect, to try to overcome the resistance rather than listen to it thoughtfully. It is easy to imagine how such persistence might escalate into the kind of angry push-pull so well known to many parents of adolescents, rather than a supportive adult–adult conversation.

Some sensitive themes

HCPs should develop their sensitivity to the contexts for illness and support. In order to decide how to respond, Marsha needs to develop some hypotheses about the situation. Some possible themes which may be significant here:

- The illness has led to a considerable invasion of privacy for the family, through the regular home visits by the nurse. We must not assume that different family members will respond to such visits in the same way (Altschuler 1997: ch. 3). From Bethany's point of view, Marsha is an uninvited guest. Knocking on her bedroom door might have been experienced as pushing personal boundaries still further.
- The visits may serve as a painful reminder to Bethany that her father is ill with further deterioration expected. It is possible that the loud music may be a way in which Bethany tries to 'block out' these visits.

- It is also possible that Bethany does need support and actually feels 'left out' or ignored. From this perspective, the door slamming and loud music might actually be an indirect way of reminding the Macmillan nurse that Bethany exists and needs attention, although offering this is not straightforward. An important counselling skill is the capacity to tolerate ambiguity and accept that several contradictory factors at once may all be partly true. Some of the delicacy of the situation may be that Bethany both needs support while also being angry and upset that this is so.
- Bethany may feel jealous of the close relationship between her father and the Macmillan nurse, and perhaps feel guilty or upset that she cannot offer her father the same kinds of support.
- The visits from the Macmillan nurse may remind Bethany, whether consciously or not, of feelings of abandonment and betrayal relating to her parents' separation. These feelings may be particularly painful in the context of an impending loss of her father through death, which can be experienced as another form of abandonment. Bethany's feelings towards Marsha may represent a mix between feelings based on the sad reality of her father's illness, combined with other feelings 'left over' from the parental separation. This phenomenon is something that psychodynamic theorists refer to as transference.
- Bethany may already be feeling that her father has lost many abilities and is becoming a patient in need of care rather than a parent who can care for her. For Marsha to approach Bethany about her schooling, rather than Errol, might exacerbate this feeling and undermine his parental authority.

Disempowering through 'doing for'

Reflecting on what has happened, Marsha might realize that she jumped to action ('doing for') upon hearing of a concern, rather than exploring further with Errol the extent and nature of the problem, how he understood this, and how he had tried to deal with this himself. She made the assumption that Errol needed her intervention to address the problem, rather than investigating how she might empower him to take action as a concerned father. In doing so, she may have fuelled Bethany's distress about her father's illness and the way it has made him less available to her. Using self-reflexivity, the HCP may recognize that it is her own action which has caused some of the anger, and understand the anger as helpful feedback that the HCP should offer support in a different way.

Tolerating discomfort and uncertainty

In the first instance, Marsha should simply go back to Errol and explain what has happened, and might suggest: 'I think perhaps I haven't given enough consideration before to how this illness is affecting Bethany, or indeed what she makes of my visiting you like this. I'll give that some thought before I visit you next time, and maybe you and I could spend some time talking about that.' Marsha may feel uncomfortable leaving the situation 'unresolved', but she has not actually been given cues by either Errol or Bethany that they need to be 'rescued' by her or that there is a need to hurry. Exercising counselling skills effectively sometimes means knowing when not to speak or when to withdraw. A response like this makes it clear to Errol that Marsha is available to him as a resource and that she recognizes the subject may be important to him, but without making presumptions about what needs to be done about this.

On the next visit, if Errol does not raise the topic himself, Marsha might say: 'I remember that last time I was here we got talking about Bethany a bit. Is that something that we should talk about today?', offering the opportunity but empowering Errol to prioritize the support he would like.

Enumerating concerns

If Errol does want to talk further about Bethany, Marsha could support him to list the different concerns he does have ('Are there any other ways in which this has affected her?', 'Why do you think she behaves like that?'), and invite him to outline how he has already been working to support her, valuing his role and seeking to empower him by highlighting his own resources ('How have you been dealing with that so far?', and:

'Tell me, if you were well and facing this problem with one of your children, how would you deal with that?'). The focus would be primarily on empowering Errol to take action rather than acting for him:

Errol: 'Well, I think I mentioned last time the thing that does bother me is her school attendance. She skips school a lot to look after me.'

Marsha: 'How have you tried to deal with that so far?'

Errol: 'Well, I tried talking with her about it, but she just gets angry and walks off.'

Marsha: 'Are there other ways to tackle it?'

Errol: 'I suppose I should ask to speak to the school about it. I don't think she'd thank me for that, but I'm not making much headway on my own.'

Marsha: 'What would you say to the school, do you think?'

Errol: 'Well, at the moment I don't think they even know I'm ill, and I guess that would be a start. It'd be a problem shared, anyway.'

Marsha: 'Do you think there are any other ways I can support you in this?'

Errol: 'I'm not sure really, I think it's better between me and her really, but what I will do is ask if she wants to meet you sometime. I don't think she really knows what your job is.'

Marsha: 'That's fine, I'd be happy to meet with her if she wanted to. I can leave you some of the leaflets we have about our service to help you explain if you like.'

Case note 19

Ivan is a young man with AIDS apparently contracted as a result of a long-standing intravenous drug habit. He has been admitted to the palliative care unit for respite care. It is suspected that he is obtaining extra 'recreational' drugs from outside the unit. He seems to be constantly 'high', is loud and has been verbally abusive to some of the younger female nurses. Ivan has a number of friends who visit him frequently, arriving sometimes late at night and staying until the small hours of the morning. It is also suspected that they are bringing drugs in and smoking cannabis in the unit. Since Ivan's arrival at the palliative care unit, several staff have reported thefts of small items such as bags, keys and cash.

Amanda is a nurse team leader at the unit. She has been asked by the unit manager to speak to Ivan to remind him of the unit's 'ground rules'. She knows from Ivan's hospital notes that in the past he has been physically aggressive to nurses and doctors although this has not happened in the palliative care unit. Amanda arranges to speak with Ivan on his own in the interview room, which is next to the main nursing office where other staff are writing up some notes. Although this is the most private space available that day, the sound-proofing between the interview room and the nursing office is not very good, and at times Amanda and Ivan can hear staff laughing about something next door, and catch snatches of their conversation.

The talk between Amanda and Ivan rapidly becomes very heated. Ivan argues that he is being unfairly victimized because he is a drug-user and has AIDS, 'not like all those poor old dears with cancer you like looking after', and denies that he or his friends have been causing any problems. Amanda tries to remain calm and stick with the facts, but can feel herself becoming angry and upset. Unknown to the other palliative care staff, Amanda's partner is also a drug-user and has recently been diagnosed as HIV positive. Amanda has been worrying whether to have a test herself. The conversation is reminding her of arguments she has often had with her partner.

Ivan shouts angrily: 'You just have no idea what it's like, living with this, you have no fucking idea at all. You nurses, you should get to see what real life is all about, it's fucking hard. Stuck-up bitches, what do you know about real problems? I hope you get a chance to see what it's really like being ill one day, what it's like knowing you're going to die of AIDS in some stinking hole like this.' The staff in the room next door seem to have gone very quiet.

Maintaining integrity in the face of provocation

Amanda's position here is complex and difficult. She has a responsibility to support her team and other patients through assertively upholding the hospice's ground rules, and she has a right and responsibility to herself to maintain her own integrity. Ivan offers powerful challenges to these aims, yet he is clearly in distress and has significant support needs. Any staff member in this situation will experience powerful urges to fight (e.g. through verbal retaliation: 'I don't think a drug addict has got any right to lecture me about real life. You've put yourself in this position, not like most of the other patients you're complaining about') or flight ('If you're going to be like that, I can see there's no point continuing this conversation. I'll have to speak to the consultant about this and let them talk to you').

The HCP's private concerns may colour professional reactions

The issues in Amanda's personal life may also make her particularly vulnerable to Ivan's provocations, or tempt her into defensive personal disclosures in the heat of the moment which she may later regret ('Actually, I do understand better than you think. My own partner is HIV positive'). Amanda also needs to reflect carefully whether she is inadvertently 'taking out' on Ivan some unfinished business with her own partner.

Avoiding escalation

First, Amanda needs to recognize that the interaction is escalating symmetrically and interrupt this pattern. One of the most straightforward ways is to stay silent, and see what follows. Of course, Ivan may continue the tirade, but it also offers a possibility for him to calm slightly, or offer an apology, or do something different rather than continue the tit-for-tat.

Sometimes 'time-out' is needed for calmer reflection

Second, Amanda needs to consider whether she is able to continue the conversation at this time, considering her own needs and capabilities. It may be that she is too upset to continue and judges that she needs other support herself: 'Ivan, I think we're both digging ourselves deeper into a hole here. You're upset and I'm upset, and maybe we both need a bit of space to calm down a bit and think again before we try to talk more about this. I'll come back again later today and see if one of my colleagues can sit in as well to help us find a way through this.' This is congruent with her own feelings, breaks the escalation, helps her maintain her own integrity, and avoids blaming Ivan for the situation, yet assertively restates that there are some issues which the unit does need to resolve with Ivan. Amanda allows herself the possibility of using support from a colleague. This may itself be a valuable way of modelling for less experienced staff that it is acceptable to ask for help when problems arise.

There may be a temptation to placate angry patients

When faced with such anger, some HCPs may feel tempted to placate the patient, protecting themselves by submission. This temptation may be particularly marked when working with patients who have some history of violence, or who are being seen in an isolated location (e.g. an individual home visit). For instance, Amanda might reply: 'Ivan, I didn't mean to upset you. I'm sorry if I've said the wrong thing. I would like to understand better how you feel, honestly.' Although this breaks the escalation of hostility, it does not assert the rights of staff and the ground rules which protect other patients.

Accepting the patient's feelings does not mean agreeing with their behaviour

If Amanda does feel sufficiently 'on balance' to stay with Ivan, the priority is to find a way of validating and accepting the patient's emotional experience, without being bullied away from the boundaries that the unit requires. The challenge is to convey respect and interest for Ivan as a person with feelings, without condoning his behaviour: 'Ivan, I really would like to understand how this feels for you. That's how we'll be able to help you, but I can't hear what it is you're telling me when you are shouting and swearing at me . . . I also think it's important that you hear what I have to discuss, so perhaps we could take this one step at a time.'

Recognizing the validity of Ivan's feelings while remaining assertive

Another way to continue the discussion might be: 'Yes, I think you're right that I don't understand how you feel. Ivan, I really would like to try to understand better, and perhaps that would help both of us. I guess that you might be feeling frightened and isolated, and I think it is pretty clear that you're very angry. I realize you've got a lot to be angry about. I think I'm getting angry too – just like anyone else, I don't like being sworn at. Do you think we could try to talk about this again adult to adult, or would you rather do that a bit later when we've both had a chance to calm down a bit?' This does not shy away from the need to talk further with Ivan about ground rules, but does attempt to recognize the validity of his feelings, including that of feeling misunderstood. Amanda offers a congruent disclosure of her feelings, linking this with a specific behaviour of Ivan's that she wants him to change. The invitation to talk 'adult to adult' invites Ivan to take an observer position in relation to himself and reflect on other ways in which he could try to express his needs.

There is of course no way to guarantee that Ivan will accept such an invitation, but the task is to keep trying without fighting with the patient, fleeing, or losing one's own integrity. The sensitive use of good counselling skills cannot ensure agreement and progress in all cases, but it does increase the possibility for a meaningful dialogue.

Main learning points

- The idea that patients may be angry with us, or us with them, may not be easy to reconcile with our self-images as caring professionals. However, we need to recognize that anger is an understandable and common reaction to the dilemmas confronting all those dealing with serious illness.

- It is easy for the frustration that we feel when things are not going well to slip into an escalating cycle of anger and hostility.
- Our own discomfort at anger may lead us to try to 'rescue' people or deflect anger, rather than accept it or try to understand it better.
- 'Fight or flight' are common responses to anger. In order to work therapeutically with the emotion HCPs must monitor the temptation to avoid issues which provoke the expression of anger, and must avoid retaliating 'in kind'.
- Sometimes people may be angry at us because we are doing our job or for what we represent, rather than because we are doing something wrong. Palliative care professionals need to be able to live with this dilemma, while remaining flexible in their approach.
- Anger may sometimes be fuelled by feelings inappropriately carried over from other relationships, but we must be careful not to use this as a blanket excuse to dismiss the validity of people's feelings about us.

Chapter **7**

Palliative care and children

Introduction

It is beyond the scope of this book to examine the specific issues relating to the care of children who are ill and have palliative care needs. Some useful starting points for readers who wish to explore those issues further include:

Give Sorrow Words: Working with a Dying Child, by Dorothy Judd (London, Free Association Books 1989)
Death Talk: Conversations with Children and Families, by Glenda Fredman (London, Karnac 1997)
An Intimate Loneliness: Supporting Bereaved Parents and Siblings, by Gordon Riches and Pam Dawson (Buckingham, Open University Press 2000)

This chapter focuses on the use of counselling skills in relation to families with children where an adult has palliative care needs. We use two examples to suggest how palliative care staff may use counselling skills to (a) support children trying to make sense of conflicting messages about illness, and (b) negotiate with parents how young children can be involved in their care in an in-patient setting.

Case note 20

Timothy's parents divorced when he was 5 years old. He stayed with his mother and baby sister, while his father moved into another house in the village. Three years later, his mother Angela developed lung cancer. She was admitted to the hospice twice for symptom control, once for painful coughing that exhausted her, and once to try to find ways to reduce or mask the stench of a foul-smelling sputum she coughed up copiously.

For Angela's first admission, her sister Gwynneth moved into her home to help look after Timothy and his sister Kate. Gwynneth was called away on business shortly before Angela's next admission, and with some reluctance she asked her ex-husband John to look after the two children at his house. During her stay at the hospice, John brought the children to visit his ex-wife regularly, although he tended to wait outside in the reception area rather than spend much time with Angela.

Marvin was an auxiliary nurse at the hospice. He noticed Timothy following him around the corridors. After a few days, Marvin and Timothy were quite friendly together and swapped jokes and sometimes played games together in the patients' day lounge. One morning, however, Timothy seemed in a more serious mood and said very directly and earnestly: 'Please don't let my mummy die, will you? My daddy says she's going to die and we'll have to live with him, but I don't want to. He scares me. My mummy says she's going to get well as soon as she can.'

Accepting the connection and the relationship rather than emphasizing roles

Marvin has already exercised some useful counselling skills in forming a meaningful connection with Timothy through channels appropriate for his age, such as playing games and allowing the boy to watch him at work (Herbert 1996). The development of this relationship has led to a point where Timothy trusts Marvin enough to share some very significant fears and anxieties with him unprompted. This is potentially a valuable opportunity, since Timothy may not have established similar connections with other members of the hospice team (hence Marvin should not reply: 'Timothy, that's not really for me to say – you need to ask the doctors about that. I'm just an assistant here'). However, Marvin is also faced with the delicate task of responding sensitively and empathically without losing his professional 'neutrality', and without offering inappropriate reassurance that may later backfire.

It may be tempting to change the subject

Faced with such an awkward encounter with a young boy in such distress, many of us may feel an urge to try to 'rescue' the child by changing the subject and 'distracting' Timothy: 'Try not to worry too much Timmy, we'll do our best and the doctors here are very good. C'mon, lets have another go on the Playstation.' While this does not fuel conflict or disempower the family, and lets the HCP 'off the hook', it squanders the opportunity to use Timothy's approach therapeutically.

We may also recognize that such replies can reflect a desire to rescue ourselves from a distressing discussion. In a culture which emphasizes the vulnerability of childhood (das Gupta 1994), HCPs may find these urges to rescue and/or avoid such situations particularly marked when dealing with young children.

It is a mistake to take sides when young children are caught in the middle

There may be a temptation to offer reassurance by 'taking sides' between Timothy's mother and father. Since Marvin will know Angela relatively well, and since Timothy is expressing some hostility and fear towards his father, Marvin may be tempted to say something like: 'Timothy, I don't know what's going to happen with your mum, but I'm sure no-one would make you live with someone who scares you. What does your Auntie Gwynneth have to say about this?' This runs the risk of fuelling divisions between Timothy and his father at a time when the family is trying to find ways to work together, and is unlikely to alleviate the pressure on Timothy as a 'piggy in the middle' between his mother and father.

It is inappropriate for Marvin to offer Timothy assurances about who he will live with in the future. Marvin does not know and is not in a position to decide. For all Marvin knows, this may already be a topic of intense discussion between John, Gwynneth and Angela, and a clumsy intervention may be unsettling and undermining. Equally, it would be unhelpful to 'side' with Timothy's father at this point by confirming the prognosis: 'I'm sorry, Timothy, but I think your daddy's right. Your mum is very sick, and we can't make her better.' Although this may seem to offer Timothy honest and congruent feedback about his mother's condition, it is potentially very disempowering of Angela, and might even fuel a rift between Timothy and his mother if he feels she is simply lying to him.

Focus on feelings, offer an understanding of the dilemma rather than attempted solutions

A useful guide for HCPs faced with this kind of situation is to focus on responding to the feelings involved, and to help recognize the dilemmas rather than try to solve the problem. Timothy is clearly in a painful position receiving such contradictory messages from his parents. He is in a bind, where there are significant risks for him in accepting or rejecting either parent's position. Faced with such binds, adults may have a choice simply to 'walk away' from the conflict. This is not an option for young children who are still dependent on others for their basic care and for their emotional and psychological support. To avoid disempowering either parent, Marvin needs to maintain a non-judgemental stance towards their handling of the situation, while to support Timothy, Marvin needs to offer empathic understanding.

Naming the dilemma

For example, Marvin might reply: 'That sounds really hard, not knowing what's going to happen and feeling like people are saying different things to you. What do you think is going to happen with your mummy?' or: 'Poor Timothy, you do sound frightened. What do you think is happening?' or simply: 'How are you feeling right now?' These kinds of responses acknowledge the emotional level of the communication, and invite further discussion at this level, without trying to rescue Timothy by offering facile solutions or inappropriate reassurance.

Helping to make meaning

An honest way of validating Timothy's demand to save his mother that does not cut across either parent's coping strategy may be: 'I guess you know I can't make a promise like that. No-one can. Everyone is doing their best to help your mother feel as comfortable as possible, but you know that she is very sick,' and then inviting Timothy to remember what he has seen and heard about his mother's illness to date ('When did you first notice that your mother wasn't well . . . what happened?') and how this has affected him ('What was it like for you when the doctor came to visit . . . What did you think was happening?'). Helping the child to review his experience of the illness so far by 'telling the story' is a way of supporting him to make his own sense of the experience, while respecting the ways in which his family is already trying to work with him (Fredman 1997).

Another way to do this is to ask him about his sister's experience and understanding of the illness, since in talking about the effects on his sister Timothy may also be indirectly speaking about the issues facing him ('Does your sister understand what cancer is . . . She's quite young, isn't she? Do you think she knows what it means to talk about someone dying?').

Not feeling over-responsible

It is important that Marvin should feel able to use counselling skills to offer some therapeutic response, but without feeling oppressed by a sense that he is solely responsible for addressing Timothy's needs. It is possible that as Timothy is encouraged to share some of his feelings and make sense of the illness experience, he may express some guilty feelings about his mother's illness and his part in this. Young children will not understand the ways in which illnesses are caused or treated in the same way as adults (Altschuler 1997: ch. 5). It is quite common for children to assume they bear excessive responsibility for many events, perhaps including the illness itself (Herbert 1996).

Offering clear information in simple terms is an appropriate response to address basic misunderstandings which may cause distress (e.g. Timothy: 'Mummy started coughing after I burnt the toast in the kitchen. I think she must have breathed in too much smoke.' Marvin: 'It sounds like you might think you caused this? Trust me on this, the doctors and I know that you don't get the kind of illness your mummy has because of that kind of smoke. It wasn't your fault'). This kind of basic factual reassurance and information is highly appropriate, and for many children is enough to minimize oppressive feelings of self-blame.

However, some children may continue to be very critical of themselves in relation to the illness ('That's what Auntie Gwynneth said too, but I don't believe her. I keep dreaming about it'), and this would be a cue for Marvin to consider a referral to a more specialist resource such as a service counsellor or a Macmillan nurse with particular experience of work with children. In the first instance such a referral would need to be discussed with Timothy's parents.

Confidentiality and child protection

Working with young children in distress may sometimes present particular issues for HCPs relating to confidentiality and to the protection of children from danger such as abuse. Difficulties may arise if HCPs are insensitive to cues that children offer about problems or, conversely, if they are too ready to leap to false conclusions or ask children leading questions. When children disclose information to us that indicates they are at risk in some way, problems may be further compounded if we have mistakenly guaranteed in advance that we will 'keep the secret' (Corby 1993).

In the example above, it is unclear what Timothy means when he says that he is scared of his father. He may simply mean that it scares him when his father tries to explain how ill his mother is. At another extreme he may be hinting that his father is abusive towards him. Many other explanations are possible. Marvin could ask: 'I wasn't sure what you meant when you said that your daddy scares you. Could you say a bit more about that?' This very open question expresses interest and concern but does not 'lead' Timothy into a particular answer or pressurize him. If Timothy answers: 'No, I can't, I'm not allowed to say', Marvin should accept this but discuss further with more senior staff how this might be followed up.

If Timothy answers: 'Only if you promise not to tell anyone else', Marvin should avoid such a guarantee. Depending on the nature of the problem, it may be necessary (perhaps legally so) to involve other people. Rather than make a false promise Marvin might say: 'I won't tell anyone else unless they need to know so that we can all help to keep you safe. What is it that you're scared of?' It is important to listen carefully, keep an open mind ('It scares me when daddy cries. I've never seen him do that before'), avoid pressurizing or leading a child, and it is vital that the HCP should feel able to seek advice and support from other team members. All health care organizations should have policies regarding the management of confidentiality and issues relating to children, and HCPs need to be mindful of these.

Working with young children may pose a substantial emotional burden

Working with young children in palliative care can impose a substantial emotional burden on the HCP. While it is constructive to use the relationships that develop naturally with children and certain staff members, it is important that this is not exploited by other staff in order to avoid dealing with children's distress. Children should not be encouraged to become over-reliant on one team member, who will of course only be present for certain shifts, and have other patients to deal with. This may mean that other team members will have to make a point of trying to form connections with the child, perhaps through initial introductions and shared activities involving the team member who has made the first connection.

HCPs must remain mindful that they may represent many aspects of the health care system to the child, above and beyond the relationship that they have tried to provide. It is not uncommon for children to become very angry with a staff member they have been close to before their parent's condition deteriorates or they die. Children may feel badly let down by the palliative care team in general, and in particular by HCPs that they have come to know personally.

Case note 21

For much of the day the men's ward of the hospice was a quiet place, with the mumble of a TV in the background, fitful snores, and quiet conversations with visiting relatives. However, Jack's children were young and noisy and came visiting most evenings with their mother Evelyn. While Jack and Evelyn sat and talked, the three children played games and chased round the corridors of the hospice. Sometimes Jack smiled and chuckled as they hurtled by.

At first the staff experienced the noise of young children as a breath of fresh air and a reminder of vigorous new life amidst all the illness they worked with. However, it became apparent that the children were if anything getting more rather than less exuberant in their play each time they visited, and other patients began to complain. Several patients commented that it was difficult to get much rest or to relax with the noise which added to their fatigue, while others complained that they felt unsafe trying to walk around the corridors in case the children knocked them over.

Staff nurse Arthur went to raise this with Jack and Evelyn during one visit, asking if they could keep the children by their bedside and quieter on visits. Evelyn and Jack looked irritated, and Jack said: 'They're just kids aren't they, kids will be kids after all. Let them be.'

Hypothesizing to empathize with the patient's perspective

Arthur and the team need to develop some hypotheses about the situation in order to offer an approach that is not simply an authoritarian enforcement of 'house rules'.

- Reflecting upon their own feelings about the children, staff may consider whether the children represent something very valuable to Jack and his wife about life and health, balancing the many losses they are experiencing. Jack's apparent pleasure in the children's antics is a powerful hint towards this, and is of course a possible encouragement to the children to do 'more of the same'. His smiles and chuckles will be feedback that they are helping to cheer up their unwell father. It is also quite possible that the children have been getting similar messages from some staff members welcoming the distraction from the sadness and routine of working life on a ward dealing with serious illness.
- In accepting in-patient care, patients open themselves to many additional losses such decreased choice and autonomy about their routines, their meals, their privacy, etc., and a loss of familiar and comforting cues from the home environment. Arthur's request may be experienced as a demand for Jack to surrender even more independence.
- There may be a clash between the culture of the ward and the culture/background of the patient. It is possible that what some other patients and staff see as unruly behaviour seems entirely unremarkable to Jack and his wife. Nonetheless, simply remaining non-judgemental seems problematic since other patients are being disturbed.
- Evelyn and Jack may have been discussing another important issue, and resent the uninvited interruption.
- The couple may feel angry that they are being 'told off' in the hearing of other patients and are defensive because of this.
- Either or both of the couple may well feel very fatigued or worn-down already. Fatigue is a much under-recognized symptom affecting many palliative care patients. It is possible that Evelyn and Jack are already conscious of the issue, but feel too exhausted to control the children assertively. Arthur's

approach may seem like yet another potential drain on Jack's energies.

- Evelyn and Jack may be aware of the issue already but feel annoyed that this is being presented as their problem rather than one relating to the ward's childcare facilities (or perhaps to a lack of childcare support offered by other family members). Young children may well feel bored and unstimulated by many healthcare environments designed for adult patients.
- The children and/or their parents may be unused to spending much time together as a quiet group, and in particular may not know how to talk with each other in the context of illness.

Hypothesizing like this can be a useful way to help staff develop an empathic understanding of a situation, which in turn can help staff approach problems such as this from the patient's perspective. If this is not done, the situation may well develop into a straightforward confrontation with the family ('I'm sorry Mr Smith, but rules are rules and we have to think of the other patients too. We've been getting complaints and it can't go on like this'). Since the patient is vulnerable and dependent on the HCPs, this 'battle' would probably be won by the organization, but sowing the seeds for much poorer collaboration and lack of trust in future care. Evelyn and Jack might feel angry, humiliated and/or guilty.

Collaborating rather than opposing

More constructively, Arthur might continue: 'I appreciate it can be difficult for any young children in a ward like ours which doesn't have much for them. I wondered if we might be able to talk about that a bit to see if there are ways that we can help them to feel welcome here without disturbing other patients too much. I'm sorry if I sounded critical. It's just that some of the patients here can get very tired, so we need to balance helping you and your family feel at home with making sure everyone can get the rest they need. I'm sorry if I haven't picked a good time to raise this with you. We could discuss it later if that would be better for you both?'

This conveys respect for couple's rights to private time

together while asserting that this is something which needs to be addressed for other patients' benefit. Choice is offered about the timing for further discussion. Some recognition is offered that the conditions may be difficult for any family in this position ('normalizing'), rather than blaming Jack and Evelyn as bad parents. Arthur accepts a share of responsibility to do with the environment. The references to 'feeling at home' and to other patients' fatigue provide possible invitations to share Jack's own experience. Taken as a whole, this approach offers a collaboration with the parents to support their children, rather than an opposition against them.

Valuing the patient's authority as a parent

If the invitation to discuss the problem is accepted, then a further constructive avenue is to express curiosity about the approach that the parents believe will be most effective: 'We're aware that some of the other patients do feel nervous when the children start running. Obviously, as their parents, you know the children best. Do you have any ideas how we could start to address this?' and: 'Are there any ways that we could help you to do that?' This restates the staff's concern clearly, but invites the parents to use their expertise and authority in relation to their own children.

Wondering what the children may be asking for

It is possible that the children's 'noisiness' can be heard as a reminder to everyone that they may also have support needs which require further attention. This could be constructively discussed as a 'normal' issue in the context of serious illness rather than a failing of Jack and Evelyn. If the parents suggest that the situation is unfamiliar to them and the children's behaviour very novel, the focus might switch to helping them to make meaning out of these changes ('You said that the children have never been in a hospital before. Tell me, what have you said to them so far about their father being here . . . Do the two of you agree what needs to be said to them, or are there aspects where either of you are less sure what to say?'). A conversation about the children's behaviour can support further discussion about the children's understanding and feelings, and the way that the family as a whole is organizing around the illness.

Main learning points

- It is usually unhelpful to 'take sides' when children are caught in the middle between conflicting concerns or coping strategies of parents or other family members. The HCP must be careful to maintain a therapeutic neutrality rather than impose solutions.
- Helping children to reflect on their experiences of the illness can help them 'make sense' of what is happening. This is a valuable supportive role in its own right.
- Children's capacity to understand the causes and effects of illness will be different from adults', because of their more limited experience, and because younger children's cognitive skills are less developed. Many children experience feelings of guilt in relation to a family illness and assume that they bear some responsibility. HCPs may be able to help by offering basic factual information and reassurance.
- HCPs must be careful not to make promises of 'secrecy' to children which could compromise child protection and lead to children feeling further betrayed. Team confidentiality is not the same as secrecy. HCPs must ensure they are familiar with organizational policy relating to confidentiality, and should consult with colleagues if they have concerns.
- The emotional burden of working with young children in palliative care should not be underestimated. Teams must offer support to colleagues who are involved, and be careful not to encourage children to become over-reliant on any one team member.
- When children's behaviour presents difficulties for the team or other patients, a respectful and collaborative approach with the parent(s) is needed to value their continuing authority over their children and avoid disempowerment.

Chapter 8

Dying and death itself

Introduction

Death and dying are central themes in palliative care, although this may not mean that they are the most difficult or stressful issues for patients and carers. Palliative care professionals may sometimes be tempted to over-romanticize the idea of a 'good death'. Conversely, they may become so familiar with the routine occurrence of death in palliative care that they fail to recognize the unique nature of every death.

This chapter examines the use of counselling skills in three different situations: one in which a patient is terrifyingly aware of their imminent death, a second in which one patient's death directly affects another, and a third in which a relative becomes increasingly distressed as their partner nears death. In selecting these examples, we want to emphasize that many different people will be affected by a death and each have their own support needs.

Case note 22

Heather had finished reloading Mrs Anderson's morphine pump and was about to leave the room. Mrs Anderson had an oesophageal tumour which made it hard for her to eat or drink, and had lost a lot of weight, but she seemed comfortably settled this morning.

As Heather reached the door, she heard a retching noise, and turned to see Mrs Anderson vomiting over the bedclothes. Heather saw that the vomit was the bright scarlet of arterial blood. Mrs Anderson was white and shaking, eyes wide with fear. After a few seconds, she was sick again, blood now soaking the sheets and staining the dark green blankets. The nurse realized that Mrs Anderson was bleeding copiously from an artery eroded by the tumour, and probably had only minutes to live.

Mrs Anderson stared at Heather and asked: 'What's happening, what's happening to me? Am I dying?' She coughed up more blood.

What can Heather do for Mrs Anderson?

Many patients receiving palliative care die while asleep or while unconscious. However, there will be times when patients are awake and aware of changes signalling a rapid and potentially terminal change in their condition. Are counselling skills relevant at such times? Perhaps not if we think about such skills strictly in terms of verbal technique, or as a technical exercise. However, let us take seriously the idea that counselling skills are about an intentional use of relationship to support another person in distress.

What can Heather do for Mrs Anderson? Heather cannot help Mrs Anderson to live longer. Heather cannot solve any problems for Mrs Anderson, or help her make choices or plans. There may be no time to invite in family or friends. Although some hospices might have injections of sedatives kept nearby for such occasions, it is far from clear whether such drugs take effect quickly enough to offer benefit, or indeed whether rapid sedation is actually helpful. For some patients a loss of clarity might compound their fear through confusion.

Instead of asking what Heather can *do for* Mrs Anderson, we can ask instead how Heather can *be with* Mrs Anderson. In order to consider this question, we must use empathy to guide us. Heather will not be able to know from Mrs Anderson afterwards whether she 'did the right thing'.

Abandonment

We can imagine that it would be unhelpful to abandon Mrs Anderson in this time of final crisis. Such abandonment might come about if Heather leaves the room to seek help or perhaps to find a relative who is elsewhere in the building. By the time she returns, Mrs Anderson may well be dead. If help is needed, or if a relative must be summoned, Heather should use the patient's buzzer. Note that Mrs Anderson's fear and distress might be aggravated by Heather shouting out loudly or panicking herself. In order to support Mrs Anderson, Heather needs to help contain her own distress or panic.

There are of course other more subtle ways to abandon patients as they die. For example, Heather might busy herself trying to mop up the blood and reposition Mrs Anderson so she does not choke, or in administering a sedating dose. The point is not so much that these would be entirely inappropriate actions, but rather that in a flurry of activity to deal with the mess it would be possible to avoid the stark fact of relating to a person present and dying.

False reassurance

It may also be tempting to offer some false reassurance to the patient: 'No, don't worry, Mrs Anderson, it's nothing to worry about. Just try to be still and stay calm, and you'll feel better soon.' Perhaps if the patient could really believe this, it might be comforting, but it flies in the face of the bloody evidence. This would be highly incongruent, and the very opposite of helping patients to 'make meaning'. There is no benefit in adding confusion to fear. We might argue that we have no right to deny a patient an awareness of their fate, particularly if they have asked so directly. We cannot know what final preparation or prayer a patient might want to offer.

Heather could seek to acknowledge and validate the patient's experience, and help Mrs Anderson make sense of what is happening. In so doing, Heather demonstrates a valuing of Mrs Anderson that continues even as she is dying. Heather might hold Mrs Anderson's hand and say: 'Mrs Anderson, I think that you are bleeding from an artery. I'm afraid I can't stop that bleeding, but if you lie on your side like this it'll be easier. I can see you're frightened, and I'll stay here with you. Relax if you can, I won't leave you alone.' It is hard to know how much a patient will take in verbally at a time like this, and a simple physical connection like holding a hand, and a simple action like wiping vomit away from the lips may be more significant. If Mrs Anderson asks again whether she is dying, Heather might add: 'Yes, you are losing a lot of blood, and we can't stop that. I think that there isn't much time left.'

Messy deaths like these can be traumatic for some staff. Sharing the experience of being with a patient like Mrs Anderson in a group debriefing, handover, or supervision can be an important way for HCPs to take good care of themselves too.

Case note 23

Kenneth was a light sleeper at the best of times, and he still hadn't really adjusted his sleep pattern to the routine of the ward. He woke one night to see curtains drawn around Frank's bed, while nurses came and went with washbasins and towels. Kenneth felt sad for Frank who had problems with his bowels. The nurses had given him an enema and it seemed to have done its job rather too well; poor Frank had been incontinent at least four times that day. Kenneth had come to know and respect Frank during their time together in the ward. He felt they'd developed a common bond not just because they had the same illness, but also through shared memories of war-time experiences. Kenneth hoped the diarrhoea would stop soon. He knew that it embarrassed Frank deeply.

Kenneth turned over and dozed off again. At around 3 a.m. he awoke again. This time he saw Frank's wife Mary and his two sons, Alistair and Matt. Mary was sobbing as Alistair put his arm around her shoulder. Kenneth could hear a strange noise coming from the direction of Frank's bed, a kind of 'raspy bubbling'. He wondered what it was. Kenneth had spent some time talking to Mary and the boys when he had no visitors of his own, and felt sorry for them. He wondered what was happening.

When Kenneth awoke the next morning and looked across at the opposite bed space he felt confused. Frank's bed and locker were stripped bare and empty. He waved to a passing nurse, Gary, and asked where Frank was. Gary replied: 'We've moved him to the side-room, Ken. He had a bad night.' A little later that day Kenneth decided to visit his friend in the side room. However, when he approached the open door of the room he saw nothing but a bare room and a few white bags marked 'patient's property'.

Gary returned a little later with the trolley for the midday drugs round. With a mixture of anger and apprehension, Kenneth asked: 'What's happened to Frank? He's not in the side-room like you said.'

Recognizing the connections that patients may form with one another

It is important for HCPs to consider the relationships and attachments that patients may form with one another, especially in an in-patient context. Palliative care and family systems medicine have rightly promoted the experience of family members as an important focus for holistic palliative care. However, it is still easy for us to overestimate the significance of the professionals' relationships with patients and under-estimate the bonds that form between patients who may feel adrift in the same boat in a stormy sea. The treatment and progress of one patient may be used by another patient as a way to reflect on their own condition. Although Gary may not know that Kenneth and Frank had formed a close relationship, he should be mindful that the death of one patient may have important and immediate implications for others.

Professional-centred defensiveness versus patient-centred sensitivity

Faced with Kenneth's challenge, Gary might feel guilty, angry, or perhaps puzzled if he actually does not yet know that Frank has died. Attending to our own emotions and taking these into account in responding is a key counselling skill. If Gary feels guilty, he might recognize a temptation to reply rather defensively: 'Oh sorry, I was going to come and tell you. It's been such a busy day,' or: 'Oh, we didn't want to upset you. I'm afraid that Frank has died.' These responses demonstrate an attempt at professional-centred self-protection by excusing or shifting blame for poor communication, but do not offer a supportive response to Kenneth.

Of course, it may have been a very busy day indeed and perhaps Gary has genuinely not had time to speak to Kenneth before. A genuine but supportive initial response might then be: 'Kenneth, I'm afraid that Frank died this morning,' and: 'I'm sorry I wasn't able to let you know earlier. It sounds like that's come as a shock to you?' or perhaps: 'I should have realized that you would have wanted to know. I'm sorry.' Although these replies may not seem very different, the point is that they offer some acknowledgement of the potential impact on Kenneth, and offer him a respectful apology for the way in which he learned of Frank's death (patient-centred), rather than an excuse for this (professional-centred).

Suppose Gary doesn't know what happened?

Gary might not be aware what has happened to Frank. A poor response would be simply to reply: 'I don't know, Kenneth. I've been off the ward for a while. If you ask the other nurse, she might know.' This implies a lack of concern for Kenneth's feelings, and also carries a suggestion that team members may not communicate well or may not be very concerned about the fate of their patients. The issue is not simply how Kenneth feels he is being treated, but also what is being communicated about the value and significance of Frank's life and his death. These subtle and unintended meanings may be missed by inattentive HCPs in robust health, but to patients acutely aware of their own vulnerability it is crucial to feel that staff are interested and caring.

Only a small change would be required for a more caring answer: 'I'm sorry I don't know, Kenneth, I've been off the ward for a while. I'll ask the other nurse and come straight back to you as soon as I've finished this drug round. You do sound worried about him.' This offers a supportive action ('doing for') on behalf of the patient, combined with an empathic reflection of his concern.

Is there time to talk? Quality rather than quantity

Gary needs to weigh up whether he is able to offer a more extended conversation and discussion with Kenneth straightaway, or whether to offer to return later. If Gary must continue with the drugs round promptly, it would be unhelpful to encourage a long conversation on the spot but then rush this. Part of being congruent means not offering something which the HCP is not really in a position to provide. It is unrealistic to assume that every situation can be dealt with through lengthy conversation. Instead, we need to ensure that even brief interactions show sensitivity and understanding, and leave the door open for a continuation at less hectic times.

There is a considerable difference between: 'I am sorry about that Kenneth, I didn't really know you knew each other well. Excuse me, I have to move on so I can get the drugs out to the others now,' and: 'I am sorry, Kenneth. I realize that this has upset you. I need to get on with the drugs round now, but if it's alright by you I'd like to come back after that so we can talk a bit more about Frank. Would that be OK?'

Case note 24

David hadn't eaten or drunk for six days. He lay in his side-room at the hospice with his back to the door, eyes half-open but vacant, a gaunt figure. His breathing was changing, noisier at times, then with short spells of silence when it almost seemed as though he had forgotten to take the next breath.

When Edna arrived at 9 p.m. for her night-shift as a staff nurse at the hospice she noticed that unusually David was alone in the room. Most evenings his wife Anya sat beside him in the dim light, knitting on her lap but her fingers still. Edna heard a pronounced rattle in David's breathing, and murmured quietly: 'Not long now, David,' as she walked on down the corridor.

As she neared the staff changing room, she noticed Anya in an armchair in the patients' day lounge, alone and crying, and went in to see her.

Anya looked up quickly as Edna approached, blurting out: 'I just can't bear to be in that room with him any more, but I'm frightened to go home too. I can't leave him and I can't stay. What can I do?' and dissolved again into a flood of tears.

We may become too complacent about 'peaceful' deaths

It is sometimes possible for experienced palliative care staff to forget for a while how stressful the period for death can be for relatives. After witnessing many deaths, staff may actually come to experience a certain satisfaction providing effective care for patients who are dying and perhaps look forward to the death of a patient – not through lack of feeling or ill-wish, but through their regard for the patient's journey. It is useful to remind ourselves that even where a 'peaceful' death seems in prospect, this may not lessen the impact for the family. A death which takes several days may seem extremely 'easy to manage' for professionals while being very difficult to manage emotionally for relatives.

How can we understand Anya's position?

Exercising an empathic sensitivity about Anya's situation, Edna will be aware that Anya may be feeling tired by her long vigil, during which David will have been increasingly unresponsive and visibly 'slipping away'. Edna might also wonder whether Anya has now noticed the same death-rattle Edna heard, and how Anya understands this. Faced with this situation, Edna has two main tasks. First, to bear witness to the depth of feeling involved, expressing an empathic regard for Anya's predicament. Second, she can offer active but non-judgemental support to Anya to consider what her options are at this time (taking Anya's question: 'What can I do?' not simply as an expression of distress, but also as a request to help her make sense of this unique situation). This involves helping to clarify what Anya thinks is happening, and empowering her to make meaningful choices.

Disempowering by taking charge

It would be disempowering to 'take charge' of Anya at this point and make the decision for her, although it might offer some temporary relief to both women if Edna simply tells her what to do: 'Anya, if you feel like that it's probably best if you go home and get some rest. I think you've been a great comfort to him, but at this stage he probably doesn't even know whether you're there or not. I'll phone you if anything happens.' (Or the opposite: 'Anya, you're nearly there love. If you can stay with him just a little more, I don't think it'll be long now.')

Abandonment by remaining aloof

Anya may already be feeling very alone and abandoned, having to make important decisions on her own without the support of her partner. If Edna feels unsettled by Anya's evident distress, she might retreat into a detached professionalism which maintains her own equanimity but leaves Anya feeling even more unsupported: 'I'm sorry Anya, I don't think that's for me to say. No-one else can tell you what the right thing is to do.'

Support through being alongside another

There are times when empathy can be offered simply through the physical presence of being with someone, rather than trying to talk with someone or doing something for them. It is possible that the first response to Anya should simply be to sit with her while she cries, and perhaps to offer physical contact by extending a hand. The use of touch is a complicated and potentially powerful way of connecting with another human being, and should be used very sparingly and with careful thought to possible misinterpretations. However, it would be a mistake to assume that counselling skills are simply a matter of verbal technique. Words are only one of many ways in which we can offer something of ourselves to others.

What does Anya think is happening?

Edna (listening for a pause in the tears): 'You've been waiting with him a long while now, and it sounds like that's really hard to bear, so hard that you don't know if you can stay with him in the room any more. Do you feel that something is changing now?'

Anya: 'There's that noise now, that terrible noise – it sounds like he's choking, I just can't bear it.'

Edna: 'Yes, his breathing has changed, I noticed that as I walked past his room. That doesn't mean that he's uncomfortable or choking, it often happens when someone is as weak as your husband is now' ['doing for' by offering limited but reassuring factual information about the death rattle (Nuland 1993)].

Exploring options with Anya

Anya faces an unbearable choice between staying and going. Edna cannot make the decision for Anya, but she can help Anya feel that either of these decisions are potentially valid. Counselling skills may help in two ways. First, clarifying what Anya's worst fears are about these choices. Second, exploring whether there are possible compromises which Anya has not yet considered: 'We'll do what we can to help you. You said that you don't know whether you can bear to stay in the room with him. I wonder if I could ask what you meant by that?' If Anya replies that she is frightened of being alone with him when he dies, staff could offer to sit with her, or check if she has a particular fear about what might happen at the moment of his death.

Alternatively, Anya may feel strongly that she does not want to see him die. Edna may have a role in offering 'permission' for this: 'Some people really don't want to watch their loved one die, that is quite normal. You've spent a lot of time with him while he's been awake, and I'm sure that was helpful. He seems quite peaceful now. If you like, you could sleep nearby on a bed in the day lounge, without having to stay in the room with him. I'll let you know if anything changes. If you'd rather go home tonight to get some rest, I'd be happy to phone you later to let you know how he is.'

Main learning points

- Counselling skills can be relevant to palliative care even at the point of death itself if we understand our skills in terms of purposeful relationships rather than the exercise of particular techniques.
- It is important not to offer inappropriate reassurance to a patient facing death. This does not help the patient make sense of their experience or make personal preparations for death.
- Patients may form meaningful relationships with each other and place important meanings on the way one patient's death is handled by HCPs in relation to their own vulnerable position and their own mortality.
- High quality interaction with a patient is not the same as lengthy interaction. A brief, but sensitive and empathic exchange may be more helpful than a rushed attempt at an in-depth conversation (and may be all that the patient wants).
- Experienced professionals working in palliative care may become complacent about death, which is a unique experience for each individual and family.

- As patients near death, counselling skills may help carers reflect on their choices in staying with the patient or not. HCPs should remain non-judgemental but supportive in relation to this issue.

Chapter 9

Bereavement support

Introduction

Palliative care aims to offer holistic support to patients and to their social networks. When a patient dies, we must continue to care for those still living. As well as bereaved family and friends, we must be mindful of other patients' bereavement needs, and find ways to look after ourselves following the deaths of those we have cared for.

This is not a chapter on bereavement counselling. We have not attempted to outline the ongoing specialized therapy that is sometimes necessary to help bereaved people move on with their own lives. *Counselling in Terminal Care and Bereavement* by Colin Murray Parkes *et al.* (1996) offers an accessible introduction to this complex field. More academic reviews of the research and literature in this area are offered by the *Handbook of Bereavement: Theory, Research and Intervention*, by Margaret Stroebe *et al.* (1992), and *On Bereavement*, by Tony Walter (2000).

Instead, we use three examples in this chapter to illustrate the use of counselling skills when bereavement issues demand sensitive handling at a particular moment. While this may seem a rather limited aim, the effective handling of such occasions is a necessary complement to more specialist support.

Case note 25

The day-care group at the hospice provided an opportunity for patients still living at home to come together in a group facilitated by a nurse, an occupational therapist and volunteers, taking part in activities such as group discussion, aromatherapy, relaxation and artwork.

Albert had been the life and soul of the day-care group which met each week on Wednesdays at the hospice. He had motor neurone disease and had been confined to a wheelchair with very little strength or movement in his hands or neck for over a year, and was highly dependent on others for his physical care. However, he was always in great humour, cracking jokes and being supportive of other group members when they were feeling particularly down. Somehow, when Albert was around, everyone felt brighter.

On the last Wednesday of November, the group had agreed to talk together about plans for Christmas, and how to decorate and celebrate this within day-care. Albert was missing from the group at the start of the day, and everyone agreed to postpone the discussion until after lunch in the hope he would turn up. Frances, the nurse in charge of day-care, made some phone calls to try to find out where Albert was, as she knew that a volunteer driver had gone out to pick him up from his home that morning. Eventually a message arrived from the Volunteer Coordinator, to say that Albert had suffered a heart attack in the car on his way to the hospice and had been taken straight to the local hospital by the volunteer driver. He was dead on arrival.

Frances returned to the day-care group, where the eleven patients were talking and laughing together before lunch. As she entered the room, the patients caught sight of her face and the laughter died away. One of them asked her: 'Is it Albert? Where is he? What's happened?' One of the other patients threw down her knitting and shouted angrily: 'Oh, what's the point!'

Bereavement is not just a family matter

Holistic healthcare is not simply about caring well for individuals. It also requires us to attend to the social networks of patients who will be affected by the patient's illness and the way this is managed, including the patient's death. Most hospices emphasize their interest in supporting families and carers as well as patients, and this underpins the rationale for many bereavement support services offered to relatives. However, it is also important to consider other social networks besides the family. In particular, patients will similar illnesses may form strong connections to one another through formal health facilities and/or 'informal' organizations such as community self-help groups and survivors' organizations.

The death of a patient may mean many things to other patients

The death of one patient may be an important experience for others for a variety of reasons, such as:

- the deceased patient may have been a significant social support or contact in their own right;
- the patient's death may remind others of their own mortality and their own prognosis; and/or
- the manner of the patient's death and the way this is managed by HCPs may provide a guide to how other deaths will be supported and acknowledged.

   All of these may be relevant in considering the support needs of the day-care group in response to Albert's death. Hypothesizing about Albert's particular position or role in the group, his death removes a potent source of hope and vitality which he helped to represent for others. Adding to the sensitivity of the occasion is the timing of his death, shortly before such an emotionally charged time of year, without cues which had allowed others to say goodbye.

   Faced with this situation, Frances may be tempted to continue as though little has happened, perhaps simply to share the news factually, then to encourage the group to continue with the Christmas planning after lunch. While this task-oriented approach might be intended to convey a pragmatic message that 'life goes on', it fails to allow space for the group to process and make sense of their loss, and may also inadvertently suggest that staff are unaffected or uncaring about the lives of individual patients. It also does not make use of Albert's death therapeutically for the other patients. After all, a significant reality they are facing is that life does *not* simply 'go on'.

The response of Frances and the staff

Of course, the other staff in day-care will also have come to know Albert well. They will be affected by Albert's death, and will also have an important role to play in supporting the patient group. It could be argued that Frances should have begun by sharing the news with her staff team and agreeing their approach, rather than entering the room so grim-faced. Although this was congruent with her own immediate feelings, it may not have been the best way to engage her own team. This might also have enabled Frances to acknowledge and process her own reactions, so that when she breaks the news, she is available to meet patients' needs rather than be preoccupied with her own response.

Hearing the first reactions

More constructively, Frances should first aim to acknowledge and validate the group's expression of despair and futility. For example, after replying: 'Yes, I have some sad news about Albert. Can we sit together for a few minutes, and I'll tell you what I know,' she might then invite each member of the group in turn to say something about their own feelings. A key skill would be to remain non-judgemental in relation to these comments. For example, it would be unhelpful to dispute or challenge any expressed feelings of despair or hopelessness. Frances might also want to share something of her own feelings. Such self-disclosure would be a genuine way of conveying a respect and valuing of Albert, and a communication that staff relate to patients as people rather than as cases.

Marking the death versus continuing with the present

Frances might feel tempted to suggest changes to the day's pro-gramme, such as a cancellation of the afternoon's Christmas plan-ning. However, bearing in mind the importance of empowering patients, this should be offered as a genuine choice to patients rather than imposed because Frances feels it would not be fitting. Conversely, it would be unhelpful to impose the standards of others, for example by the guilt-inducing: 'Albert wouldn't want us to give up on Christmas; for his sake, we should get on with the plans.'

Frances might say: 'I realize this has come as a shock to all of us, and it may take some time to sink in fully. We were planning to think about Christmas after lunch. I don't know whether you still want to do that or not, or whether we should leave that for another day. After lunch let's see how people feel about that.' Instead of making the choice for the patients, Frances names and describes the dilemma that the living always face after a death – how to con-tinue in their own lives, without ignoring what has happened.

Responding to a bereavement is a process that takes time, for both staff and patients. Although there may be value in an initial response such as that outlined above in which people are invited to express their reactions, Frances and her team should avoid trying to 'compress' their bereavement support into a one-off session. Patients will have been affected to different degrees, and patients will have different needs about the degree and pacing for talking further about Albert.

The paradox of treating every death as both special and ordinary

Frances might want to suggest to the group that they consider some way of marking Albert's death or saying their own farewells to him, for example, toasting him at the end of their meal together (Imber-Black *et al.* 1988). However, this may be inap-propriate if this is not a 'tradition' generally observed in the group. Have staff or patients suggested any such rituals for other patients who have died? There is a risk that if Albert's death is singled out for special treatment because he was so popular and such a 'positive' influence in the group, that this implicitly passes a negative judgement on other patients who adopt a less cheerful approach to their illness.

It follows from this that rather than respond to Albert's death as a one-off because he was someone special, it is healthier for palliative care staff to acknowledge that all deaths are significant, with this reflected in the organization's regular processes or rituals. For example, the day-care centre might open a 'guestbook' for all patients who spend time with the group. Each time a patient dies, those that remain could be reminded that they are welcome to write a farewell comment in the book if they wish. Our point here is not to prescribe a particular kind of ritual, whether this be remembrance squares in a quilt, pages in a memory book, or plants in a remembrance garden. Rather, we are suggesting the need to offer an equality of response regardless of our personal liking or disliking for a patient, that offers fellow patients flexible ways to mark a death should they wish.

Case note 26

Carol and Tim are a young couple who recently married. Tim's mother, Mrs Treacher, died in the hospice at the weekend. Tim and his wife have returned on the Monday to collect the death certificate and Mrs Treacher's belongings. In the meeting with the administrative officer and Andrea the nurse, Carol is very polite and appreciative of all the care that her mother-in-law received.

Tim, however, seems very grim-faced and quiet. He is restless throughout the meeting, and it becomes apparent that he is agitated and angry. When his wife tries to involve him in the discussion, he comments bitterly that he doesn't see why he should be grateful, since he believes that his mother was 'Put down like a dog. She died after the doctor gave her that injection – he said it was to make her more comfortable – he didn't say it would kill her! I want to know how to make a complaint, I'm going to the lawyers about this, about all of it. I want to see all her notes, I do.'

Anger as a common reaction to bereavement

Anger is a very common element in many people's reaction to a bereavement, and may be fuelled by several factors. Sometimes the anger is at least partly founded on real errors that have been made in a patient's care by professionals. Sometimes it may be a disguised way of expressing guilt about the care that the angry person provided to the deceased.

Bad things can happen to good people

Anger may also simply be a very natural, normal response to a tragic, 'unfair' loss. For many people, one of the hardest lessons of palliative care and terminal care is simply that bad things can happen to good people, and those that we love may leave or 'abandon' us through death whether we are 'ready' for this or not.

Don't pit couples against one another

When working with couples it is always important for the HCP to avoid undermining the couple relationship. In this instance, there might be a temptation for Andrea to defend herself (and her organization) by appealing to Carol's more 'reasonable' position: 'Carol, you don't see things that way, do you? I suppose it's only natural you're more upset, Tim, as it was your mother,' or: 'Your wife seems to think quite differently.' This would be a way of being very judgemental about Tim, and which might begin to undermine one of his most supportive relationships at a particularly demanding time. This way of responding to anger is just as unhelpful as diverting blame against other team members ('Oh I am sorry, doctors aren't very good at explaining these things sometimes').

Don't argue with bereaved relatives

Anger is an understandable and natural response to bereavement for some people. The emotion itself needs acceptance and validation, rather than disputation. An argumentative response such as: 'The injection didn't kill her, it was a painkiller to settle her' is likely to provoke further anger as Tim feels unheard or, worse, accused of lying or stupidity. Of course, there may also be a sense in which Tim is right, if the painkiller was given with the primary intention of relieving pain, but had secondary effects which hastened death through respiratory depression, etc. It is possible that this scenario reflects some poor prior communication which had not adequately informed Tim about his mother's treatments.

Don't use bureaucracy as a defence

Tim has asked to see his mother's notes. Whether or not the staff feel that an error has been made with the patient's care, it is important to respond to this positively and readily – a kind of 'doing for' which does not pass judgement on his feelings or suspicions. It would seem bureaucratic and defensive to reply: 'You can't see her notes – I'll need to ask the doctor first', which also implies that the nurse values the doctor's feelings more than Tim's. A more helpful and positive response would be: 'I am sorry. I know it's awful, and I guess there's not a lot I can say to make it better. I'm happy to go through the notes with both of you if it would help. Would you like to do that now?' A powerful emotion like anger may also be a way in which other thoughts and feelings are being expressed less directly. This could be explored through an open and invitational question such as: 'Do you have other concerns we should go through?'

The aftermath

Tim may at some point feel embarrassed or guilty for becoming angry. This possibility will be reduced if the HCP accepts Tim's concerns as valid and understandable from the outset, rather than criticizing him for the way he has expressed himself. Of course, Tim may remain angry and distressed at the care that was provided. It is important that HCPs working in palliative care should not feel dependent on gratitude and praise from patients and relatives for their job satisfaction. Many people will not feel grateful in any way that we had some role in the death of one of their loved ones.

Case note 27

Amanda was a nurse team leader at the hospice. She was not surprised when a number of staff chose to attend Mrs East-erman's funeral service – she had been a popular patient with a long stay at the hospice who had died a messy and frightening death. Amanda realized that many staff felt quite deeply affected by the loss and wanted to mark this in some special way.

However, Amanda was more concerned about Cathy's request for time off to attend Mr Arbogast's funeral. Amanda knew that Cathy had already been to the funerals of five other patients from the hospice within the last two months.

Amanda asked Cathy if she was perhaps becoming too closely involved with her work, explaining that she was concerned for Cathy's well-being and had noticed how many funerals she was attending. Cathy snapped sharply: 'Well, that's better than being a cold fish like you, isn't it? At least I care about patients like Mr Arbogast and Ivan who get a raw deal from the hospice.'

Palliative care staff are involved with many deaths. Each worker must find a way to manage their emotional responses to these multiple bereavements, which allows them to continue caring for other patients and maintain their own integrity.

At one extreme, staff may claim to themselves and others that patients' deaths do not affect them and are simply 'part of the job'. They might intellectually acknowledge the significance of bereavements, but experience little emotional response. Such detachment will make it harder to form empathic relationships with patients and carers. It may also detract from the HCP's job satisfaction, since palliative care aims to accept death and bereavement as valuable aspects of human experience, rather than a failed outcome of treatment.

At the other extreme, some staff may allow themselves to be touched by each patient's death as though they had lost a close friend or family member. This carries a major risk that those HCPs will become emotionally overloaded and compromise their care for other patients. It is also questionable whether professionals have the right to claim such an emotional attachment to most of their patients – perhaps this sometimes devalues the family's own bereavement experiences.

It seems healthier to support staff to develop some balance between these extremes, and realistic to expect that we will feel more affected by the death of some patients than others. Problems will arise within teams where different HCPs attempt to impose their own preferred 'coping strategy' on their colleagues, or 'require' that colleagues will have experienced the same level of emotional attachment to particular patients.

In the example presented, it would clearly be unhelpful for Amanda to become overly defensive: 'Just because I don't go around chasing hearses doesn't mean I don't care. I just hide it better.' This reply does nothing to support Cathy or explore her concerns further, and contains an implied rebuke against displaying feelings at work.

A response such as: 'Cathy, you know we care for all the patients the same. No patient is better or worse, and all get the same consideration,' is equally unsupportive, and deeply incongruent. It denies that patients and staff are individuals and *do* experience different feelings towards one another, and will make it harder for staff to share and examine how and why these differences arise. Amanda retaliates and judges Cathy's feelings, rather than acknowledging them and inviting further dialogue.

More constructively, Amanda might reply: 'Perhaps you're right about Mr Arbogast and Ivan. They were difficult times for everyone. I would find it helpful if we could talk about them between ourselves at first. Then if it feels right, perhaps we could see if other staff wanted to talk about them as well, to see what we can all learn from them?' This validates Cathy's concern, and accepts that Cathy may be right that the team can improve their care for future patients. It invites a conversation to explore Amanda's own support needs further without framing this as a failing.

Sometimes brevity is best

Such a response runs the risk, however, of seeming overly 'preachy' or long-winded. A non-defensive and open invitation to continue the conversation rather than 'win the argument' may be preferable: 'Tell me, what do you mean by a "raw deal"? What have you noticed?'

Main learning points

- Bereavement support is part of the holistic approach in palliative care. We need to consider the needs of relatives and close friends, other patients, and our own bereavement issues as HCPs experiencing repeated losses.
- Individuals may have a wide variety of responses to a person's death, depending on their relationship to the deceased, their personal style and history, other demands on them, and their cultural/religious background.
- Anger is a natural response to bereavement for many people at some point. Defensive or argumentative responses are unhelpful. HCPs should aim for empathic responses which acknowledge the validity of such emotions.
- HCPs should not expect or depend on gratitude and praise from relatives, given the fact that we have, in a sense, played a part in the death of one of their loved ones.
- Palliative care workers who habitually distance themselves from the effect of patients' deaths may find it difficult to form empathic connections with patients and carers, while those who repeatedly form strong attachments to individual patients run the risk of compromising their care for other patients.

Chapter 10

Caring: the privilege and the price

Introduction

It has become a commonplace to talk about the costs of caring and the vulnerability of professional carers to 'burn-out'. This is seen as a process by which people in jobs which are demanding at an emotional as well as practical level may be at risk of becoming progressively disheartened and less able to undertake their work and draw satisfaction from it. Some writers have proposed that this may occur in stages such as (a) emotional exhaustion, leading to (b) depersonalization and distancing, followed by (c) guilt at one's failure to care, with damage to self-image and further demoralization (Maslach 1981; Menzies Lyth 1988; Lederberg 1990).

Like most stage models proposing to describe complex psychological processes, this is probably rather over-simplistic. For instance, it seems reasonable to suggest that we will all have phases in which we may feel more or less emotionally available, or conscious that we are not 'doing our best'. Some movement between these different stages is probably natural rather than pathological. Nevertheless, it seems important for us to be wary of extremes of these experiences. We need to watch carefully for imbalances between these negative processes and more positive experiences in which we gain job satisfaction, feel that our 'batteries' can be recharged, and can feel we are in meaningful contact with other human beings.

This chapter offers some illustrations of common themes in palliative care which may exact a demoralizing cost, and others which might help reward us and sustain our professional caring and therapeutic optimism. We suggest that these themes are very relevant to the use of counselling skills in palliative care. If we genuinely believe that an awareness of ourselves and our capacity to relate empathically to others are essential to the caring process, it follows that we should strive to monitor possible blocks and supports which may hinder or help us in this.

We also wish to suggest that entering into therapeutic relationships with others can be very double-edged, carrying with it the possibility of hurt as well as well-being. The more that we are prepared for this risk and the more we can be honest or self-congruent about our experience, the better we will be able to protect ourselves without simply withdrawing psychologically from patients. When we do find that we have somehow 'failed' patients, an appreciation of the subtle dynamics in play may allow us to be more compassionate and less judgemental of ourselves, and so help us continue to care.

Case note 28

Abdullah the Macmillan nurse had visited Mrs McPherson at home on a handful of occasions to offer advice and support concerning problems with fatigue and nausea. She was grateful for his support, partly because she gained good symptomatic relief, but perhaps also because she was lonely and there was something about him which reminded her of her long dead son Peter.

Abdullah's caseload was very heavy and there were many other patients who needed his expertise. He was confident that the district nurses and GP would be able to care for her in the weeks that might remain to her. Abdullah felt it was the right decision to discharge her from his care, but realized this might be hard for Mrs McPherson. When he explained the discharge arrangements to her, he offered to arrange some further home visits by members of the local volunteer 'Listening Ear' service. As a tear rolled gently down her gaunt cheek, she said: 'I know you've got other patients to see, but can't you just drop in sometimes and see me? I don't just want someone to listen to me, I want to know you're still there.'

Boundaries

It can be very personally challenging for an HCP to maintain appropriate boundaries around the extent of their professional support when working with patients who are facing severe problems of chronic pain and disease, bereavement, and death. Modern health service jargon often describes care in terms of 'assessing and meeting needs', but such terminology seems inadequate faced with the ocean of need presented by a lonely bereaved mother facing death. How can Abdullah ever do enough for patients such as Mrs McPherson?

His choices are stark. Abdullah can try to view his job purely in terms of technical expertise and advice, in which case her other needs are not his concern. He might simply remind her that their initial agreement or 'contract' was only that he would visit until her symptoms were under better control. This is only possible if he ceases to relate to patients as people, and instead views each encounter as a clinical problem.

At the other extreme, he can take on the responsibility of trying to comfort Mrs McPherson and remain as fully available to her as she would like. This would put him under increasingly heavy time pressure, leading him towards burn-out, and compromising care for other patients who are just as needy. Ultimately, such pressures would lead him to fail Mrs McPherson. For example, if Abdullah responded to her request by promising he would continue to drop by, then failed to do so, this would compound the sense of abandonment and betrayal that Mrs McPherson may already be experiencing.

It is possible to care without helping

Another approach is to recognize that it is impossible to meet all needs and impossible to make things 'alright' for patients like Mrs McPherson, without pretending that this does not matter.

Abdullah can continue to care without being able to help. Without being drawn into a hopeless endeavour to 'rescue' Mrs McPherson, he can offer empathic understanding and congruent compassion. He might say: 'There's a part of me that would like to say that I will, because I have come to care about you through our meetings, and I understand that you are lonely and perhaps afraid too, and you would like me to protect you from some of that. However, I don't want to make things worse by promising you something I can't do such as visiting you regularly. Professionally, I need to care for other patients too, and that means I cannot spend as much time visiting you as you might like. I realize that you may feel disappointed or perhaps angry with me about that. I apologize for that.' While this leaves the way open for further discussion of volunteer home-visiting, or renewed contact if new needs arise, it assertively and honestly states the HCP's position while attempting to communicate a positive regard for Mrs McPherson. The HCP also attempts to reflect some of the emotions that underlie the exchange, and 'validates' possible feelings of anger rather than side-stepping these, accepting responsibility rather than shifting the blame onto a third party such as 'management'.

The pain of unmet need may not mean we have failed

Relating to patients as people allows the possibility of sensitive emotional connection in this way, but also exposes us to the pain of unmet need and problems that cannot be solved. Acknowledging this dilemma allows HCPs the possibility of separating themselves from this bind without distancing themselves from the patient ('I have been unable to meet all this patient's needs, which is sad but unavoidable' versus 'I have failed her so I am a bad professional').

Case note 29

Maxwell's shift was over and it was time for him to go home. It had been a long week with eight shifts in a row, but now he had four days off when he could relax. At least that was the idea – in practice, time at home was anything but relaxing at present, with the twins just beginning to teethe, and his relationship with Marcia at a new low after the debacle of the Christmas party.

Maxwell had spent a lot of time with Conrad, a retired merchant seaman who had been admitted a week ago. Conrad had chronic obstructive airways disease compounding complex cardiac problems. He had been admitted to the hospice from a cardiac ward where he had spent several weeks 'recovering' from very unsuccessful surgery. Conrad was expecting and hoping to die very soon, and the team thought this was likely within days. Conrad had confided to Maxwell in hoarse whispers snatched between puffs on his oxygen: 'I'm so glad I'm here now, I can die in peace. I know I'm in good hands, everyone here has been so good to me.'

The team leader was still on the phone trying to arrange cover for the New Year shifts. Maxwell lingered by the office station, half-hoping he would be asked to work more shifts. He felt he had become close to Conrad and wanted to be there when he died so that Conrad wouldn't have to die alone.

Staff may need to be needed

It seems likely that many people choose to work in health care at least partially because they want to feel needed by others (Parkes and Hinde 1982; Obholzer 1994). This seems quite natural. After all, most people have a number of reasons for choosing the work they do, some altruistic and some not. Working in palliative care and using counselling skills may be especially satisfying for people who want to feel needed. After all, much of the care that can be offered is of a relatively personal nature rather than technical, and many palliative care patients are very appreciative of sensitive support. While this may constitute one of the privileges of working in palliative care, it also creates one of the hazards. If a patient does not seem to need our presence and personal support, this may be taken rather more personally than a patient preference corresponding to the technical expertise we can offer (Speck 1996).

Over-reliance on being needed at work can cause problems

In the case note above, Conrad has offered clear feedback that he values the support the palliative care team is offering him. Conrad does not indicate that he particularly needs Maxwell rather than other staff. Maxwell's desire to remain on shift is centred around his own needs rather than Conrad's. It may be that Maxwell is partly trying to use work to avoid dealing with problems in his family life and relationships, but it is also possible that his desire to 'be there' for his patients is causing problems in his home life. 'Being there' for patients at the expense of our own lives threatens our personal and professional integrity. In order to offer holistic care to our patients, we need to have a 'whole' life ourselves. This may or may not be happy, but does need to offer balance and contrast.

We cannot assume that the cost of caring will be offset by time off work

This example also illustrates the need for service managers to avoid assuming that 'time off' is an adequate solution to carer support and professional burn-out. For some people, time away from work may be refreshing and provide informal opportunities to 'debrief' or unload with a supportive partner. For others, home-life itself may be tiring or dispiriting rather than supportive, either chronically, or through particular (family) life-cycle events such as the birth of new children, illness and family bereavements. Palliative care staff must have access to effective support systems within work hours.

Following the patient's journey until death

The frequency of death in palliative care provides a particular poignancy and power to caring. Staff may feel privileged that their job involves them with patients and families at such critical moments. However, this privilege also contains a potential pitfall, that staff may sometimes become over-focused on providing support until death, whether or not this is appropriate to a given patient. This may cause difficulties within palliative care services, for example, where dying patients are discharged elsewhere (e.g. to home) so that opportunities to follow the patient's final journey are limited, when relatives or the patient do not want professionals present as they die, or when the death of a patient to whom an HCP has become particularly attached occurs while the HCP is away from work or engaged with other patients.

Good team work, including communication about deaths and opportunities to ask questions and share experiences, is an important support measure. Where this is lacking, it will exacerbate tendencies by HCPs to focus too narrowly on their personal relationships with patients rather than include the patient's relationships with other colleagues.

Case note 30

Sandra prided herself on her sensitive use of counselling skills with the patients in the oncology ward. She contrasted her own willingness to spend time with patients, talking in-depth about their difficult feelings and upsetting family issues, with nurses such as Helen, who seemed to work 'by the clock'. Sandra felt that Helen strictly apportioned her time equally between patients, without regard to their personal styles and apparent emotional needs.

Sandra was very taken aback in the monthly team support session facilitated by the hospital chaplain when the other team members started to attack her for 'not pulling her weight' and neglecting patients. She listened aghast as the other nurses complained that Sandra often spent so much time with only one or two patients that other patients felt left out, and other staff felt they had to do more than their fair share of the ward duties.

Over-emphasis on lengthy therapeutic work

There is a delicate balance to be struck in organizational palliative care settings between individualizing patient care and offering meaningful, person-to-person relationships, and the need to
ensure that limited resources are used effectively to support many
patients. Some professionals sympathetic to 'therapeutic' care are
excited by the prospect of offering high quality psychosocial
support, but then become disillusioned when they are forced to
'compromise' their high ideals because of work-load. Some, like
Sandra, may initially fail to acknowledge the need for compromise and develop a comforting illusion of 'specialness' or superi-
ority in relation to their colleagues. This sort of position is
sometimes fuelled by a confusion between counselling as such,
and using counselling skills in the course of other work. In turn,
this can deprive other colleagues of opportunities to develop their
counselling skills, or devalue their own less prominent or briefer
work with less emotionally articulate patients.

Avoidance of therapeutic work

In contrast, other professionals may feel challenged or even
threatened by the prospect of entering into emotionally charged
relationships with seriously ill patients, and use time pressures as
an excuse to avoid forming individualized relationships with
patients. Failure to work in-depth with particularly needy patients
may then be excused on the grounds of 'fairness' to other
patients, ignoring the variety of patient need and confusing high
quality psychosocial work with lengthy work. Sometimes, emotionally demanding conversations might be 'dumped' on a team
member known to be more interested in such work, further
avoiding chances to develop skills in this area and potentially
overloading the colleague.

Acknowledging competing demands

If these tensions are not acknowledged and discussed openly
within teams on an ongoing basis, conflicts may escalate and

become very damaging as the team 'splits' along polarized lines rather than addressing a shared concern. Self-awareness on the part of individual HCPs is a valuable first step, but cannot substitute for the development of a team ethic through regular group discussion. Similarly, 'one-off' team discussions may have some value, but are unlikely to keep team members in tune with one another, particularly as staff change and develop and as clinical demands on the team change.

Case note 31

Marina was a home-care nurse with a palliative care team. She was often offered small gifts and presents by grateful patients and families, but usually she declined these politely, saying: 'That's kind of you, but this is part of my job.' However, Mr and Mrs Fincham were so insistent that she accepted a box of chocolates and a bunch of flowers after one night visit. It would have seemed churlish to refuse. The next time she visited, they gave her an even bigger bunch of flowers, and a crate of beer which their son carried out to her car. On the next visit, Mrs Fincham pressed an envelope into Marina's hands, saying: 'We want you to have this. We know he hasn't got long, and he wants to make sure he's thanked you properly. You've done so much for us already, and it's his way of saying thank you. Please don't say no.'

Accepting thanks too readily

One of the rewarding aspects of working in palliative care is the gratitude that many patients and relatives express. However, this too can be hazardous. If we are too dependent on gratitude, we may find it more difficult to establish good working relationships with patients who are not overtly appreciative or who are actively annoyed that they are ill and in need of care. Equally, we may unconsciously distort our care through efforts to attract praise and thanks, which might sometimes disempower patients from doing things for themselves, or inhibit patients from expressing how they really feel about us if they are critical of our care.

Failing to accept thanks

It follows from this that we must find ways to give ourselves credit for the good work that we do, rather than rely on hearing this from clients. We must develop self-awareness to offer ourselves honest feedback. This in turn will leave more space for clients to tell us what they really think of our care. However, an over-emphasis on this can render us unable to accept positive feedback from patients, and deny patients the normal, human action of expressing thanks. If patients are frequently in a position of having to accept things from others, it can be symbolically important for them to offer something back.

Accepting the message of a gift

In the case described, Marina may feel compromised by the escalating thanks which now seems to involve financial reward, although her acceptance of the first gift was based on an empathic consideration of the sensitivities involved. While it would reverse any therapeutic benefit from this initial decision for Marina to bluntly decline the offer ('I'm sorry, that's very kind, but I can't accept that'), it would be highly unprofessional to accept a personal financial gift. Instead it would be important to accept the *intention* of the gift, while emphasizing Marina's role as a representative of a team service ('That is very kind, I'm glad I've been able to help. I really appreciated the flowers, but I'm not allowed to accept any money personally. What I can do is get you some information on making a donation to our service if you like. Shall I do that?').

What might gifts mean besides gratitude?

Marina might also want to spend some time reflecting on the case afterwards, either on her own or in clinical supervision. What is it about this case that led to the situation developing in this way.

For example, might the increasing gifts reflect a growing anxiety shared by the couple that they will not be able to cope with Mr Fincham's death, and hence a desperation to 'hold onto' Marina? If so, this might suggest that Marina should restate her availability and continuing commitment to support on her next visit, and invite the couple to say more about their feelings that time is running short and the implications of this for them both. When presented with a gift, it is a useful discipline to ask oneself what additional meaning the gift might have besides gratitude.

Case note 32

Staff nurse Una sat with her supervisor in their monthly hour together:

Una: 'Work is horrible at the moment, morale is really low and everyone is bitching at everyone else. It doesn't help that we get inappropriate admissions of people who would be better looked after somewhere else.'

Supervisor: 'Do you have anyone particular in mind?'

Una: 'Well, Agnes is back. I don't know why they keep agreeing to give her respite admissions. She would be better looked after in an old people's home. We can't do anything else for her, and she's just so demanding. Always wanting something, but nothing we do ever seems good enough.'

Supervisor: 'Is Agnes is the young woman with motor neurone disease? (Una nods.) Hasn't she been coming to you for a few years now?'

Una: 'Yes, but she can't even talk now and she just sits there all twisted in the chair, dribbling spit from her mouth and staring . . . Apart from when she blinks of course to try to tell us if she wants or doesn't want something and trying to do that takes an eternity – time we could better spend with other patients.'

Supervisor: 'She really fires you up?'

Una: 'Well, it's no wonder. I look at her and I feel angry . . . What is she holding on for? Why does she do this to us? There can't be any quality of life for her just sitting there.'

Supervisor: 'How do you cope with that kind of frustration?'

Una: 'Well . . . it's terrible I know, and I know I should be more patient and tolerant and understanding and all that other stuff, but because she's in a side room on her own it's easier to avoid her. I mean we still go in and wash her and feed her, though we're trying to arrange volunteers to come and do that, but it's just easier not to have her in your face all the time.'

Patients who seem like intractable problems

The rewards of palliative care can seem very elusive when working with patients who have very chronic but relatively stable conditions, and who appear to others to have very poor quality of life. Many of the most challenging situations in palliative care are to be found not within the relatively high profile and well-resourced areas of cancer care and hospices, but in the regular home visits by district nurses to lonely and frightened house-bound patients, or with poorly paid care staff in unstimulating nursing homes. Although we may be able to remind ourselves intellectually that it is the patient's quality of life (not our perception of it) that matters, this may be of little comfort if the patient has very limited capacity to express themselves, or if the patient confirms our view that their experience is indeed deeply unpleasant. In these circumstances, we are faced with a lengthy and stressful journey with no end in sight and little prospect of satisfaction *en route*. If it is difficult to communicate with the patient, and there is little positive feedback offered by family members which reminds us of the humanity of the patient, it becomes easy to forget that the patient is anything other than a problem.

Empathy may make some situations harder to bear

No easy answers can be offered to these situations. If we are conscientious and reflective practitioners, our very self-awareness and capacity for empathic insight may almost make things worse, as we recognize the many shortcomings of our care and our attitude towards the patients, while retaining an appreciation of the awfulness of the patient's experience. We may be tempted to dream that some patients are 'beyond' palliative care, or can best be cared for by some imaginary agency that is anywhere other than ours.

Perhaps what can be done is to attempt an honest, congruent admission of how we feel to ourselves and to others who are supporting us (as Una is trying to do with her supervisor). Then at least we may avoid creating false expectations for ourselves, and we can monitor carefully how our dislike for certain patients may tempt us to offer care that is poor. If we cannot take the first step of admitting this is happening, we will be unable to correct our failings, and we will be unable to forgive ourselves. If we can become aware of our shortcomings while remaining non-judgemental, we may be able to change the quality of our caring, and extend compassion towards ourselves (Altschuler: ch. 8).

Main learning points

- We will not be able to meet all the needs of every patient. Professional case-load management may be upsetting for both patients and HCPs. This distress can be helpfully acknowledged, but is not itself a sign of failure.
- We must be careful not to confuse our desires to be needed or to be useful to patients, with any given patient's need for us. We must give priority to the needs of patients and their families, not our own. This requires self-insight and honesty.
- The use of counselling skills may be seen as desirable and high-status by some staff, and challenging or distressing by others. This sometimes shows in disputes about time allocation in teams. It must be addressed through ongoing discussion to ensure a sense of coherent team purpose which respects differ-

ences between HCPs while offering quality services to all patients, meeting both psychosocial and physical needs.

- Many palliative care patients and relatives offer gifts. We should consider carefully what such apparent gratitude might mean, particularly in relation to concerns about future care needs. There are pitfalls both in being too ready to accept gifts, and in being unwilling to accept thanks.

- Some palliative care situations are extremely distressing and offer few 'rewards' for anybody involved. There is much that we cannot make better however hard we try. Accepting this is one of the hardest tasks and most valuable lessons of palliative care.

- Well-developed empathic skills may make it more painful to 'stay with' such situations. Support from others is vital. Managers must not assume that such support is available outside work for all HCPs.

- Being honest with ourselves about our shortcomings is an important step in remaining compassionate and non-judgemental about ourselves.

Chapter **11**

Developing counselling skills

Introduction

In this chapter we suggest some ways in which palliative care professionals can develop their counselling skills. Some of these can be implemented by individuals interested in their own professional development, while others require more concerted or collaborative action at an organizational level. All the options discussed have costs of some sort, most obviously in terms of time and money. However, we have deliberately placed this chapter after some consideration of the price and privilege of working in palliative care. This is to emphasize that:

- sensitive work in this field offers some powerful rewards which can more than recompense the effort and energy required to enhance skills, but also that
- attempts to develop greater sensitivity to the emotional and psychological themes in palliative care may make HCPs more open or exposed to the pain inherent in their work.

We see no easy way around this dilemma, but acknowledging this may be a helpful step in understanding why we are sometimes reluctant to develop our counselling skills through the resources and measures which are available to us.

Listening to feedback from patients and carers

One of the most important ways to develop counselling skills is to listen carefully to the feedback that we get from patients and their family when we work with them. Sometimes this means that we should make a point of asking patients how they experience our work with them. However, some particular problems arise in seeking and interpreting patient feedback in palliative care. First, patients and family members with palliative care issues are generally in an extremely vulnerable state. This may mean that (a) when our support is poor, it may be quite risky for patients to express their dissatisfaction for fear of alienating us, and (b) even when our support is good, we should not expect that all patients will be appreciative. We become involved with patients because illness has crept uninvited into their lives, not because they wanted our services. Second, we will be unable to seek clear feedback from patients who are extremely weakened, and where patients have died we cannot assume that feedback from their family and friends about our care fully reflects the patient's own views.

How can we learn to listen to patients in the face of these difficulties? First, we must accept that what we think we hear from patients is a matter of interpretation, not one of certainty. At best, we can make an informed and sensitive guess about the meaning of a patient's communication, guided by our hypotheses about their current situation. In so doing, we must remain open to the possibility that we have misunderstood and be very ready to reach a new understanding. We can ask ourselves: 'What are the different possible meanings behind the patient's communication? Which of these possible meanings would be useful in guiding me to refine the care I have to offer this patient?' Second, we can take great care to avoid becoming defensive or rebuking patients when they are critical of our care, and instead welcome their communication and express a genuine curiosity to learn more. We must assume that every patient has something to teach us. The issue is whether we allow them space to tell us, and whether we are willing to hear.

Organizational and cultural factors

It would be unreasonable for us to present the development of counselling skills as a responsibility borne only by individual HCPs. Access to support such as clinical supervision, debriefing sessions and external courses will be dependent on time, money and permission from employers. However, we want to go beyond these material considerations to highlight the role of the organizational attitude or culture, and the role of institutions beyond the HCP's immediate employer.

Material considerations are only part of the story

Even where an organization is willing to provide some time and funding for staff training or supervision, this will be ineffective if staff are not supported in their attempts to use good counselling skills (for example, if other staff insensitively interrupt important conversations with patients). Similarly, staff will become demoralized if their contributions to team discussions and care planning about psychosocial aspects of care are not invited, valued and used, or are treated as an afterthought. Conversely, staff with good counselling skills may sometimes be 'over-used' by colleagues who delegate 'difficult conversations' to them since they are 'good at that sort of thing'. As with interactions between individuals, it is quite possible for an organization to give very mixed messages about the value of an approach. Securing financial resources is sometimes the least problematic issue in developing counselling skills!

We need to accept responsibility for our own contribution to the organizational culture

It follows from this that all HCPs need to be mindful of the ways in which they contribute to and shape the organizational culture. 'Top-down' influences are undoubtedly very important (e.g. a hospice consultant who insists that all team discussions of patients begin with a doctor's presentation of biomedical aspects is making a clear statement about the secondary place of inter-personal processes and the patient's subjectivity). However, top-down influences may also be mediated by 'bottom-up' and peer interactions. A nurse trying to develop counselling skills will be supported in this if her colleagues express an interest in her views and case notes, and offer feedback about positive effects for patients.

Reflecting on practice

It has become a commonplace to suggest that HCPs should reflect on their work, although simple definitions of reflective practice remain elusive (Johns 1998). Reflective practice involves spend-ing time thinking and feeling about encounters with patients, and thereby developing new understandings to guide future care. The assumption is that this will help us to do more of what works, and less of what does not. We would argue that reflection is not simply a way to develop other counselling skills but is also an important counselling skill in its own right. In practice, however, this apparently simple idea can be remarkably difficult to foster or encourage. Why might this be so?

Some biases and blocks to reflective practice

We may not realize what there is to reflect on . . .

When we try to remember an experience, inevitably our recall will be incomplete, and our memories will be inaccurate: we will 'remember' some details that are distortions or simply wrong. In particular, we will tend to recall the details of an experience that we believe were most salient. If we have been trained to attend to physical aspects of care, we may fail to notice and/or recall sig-nificant emotional and verbal aspects of a situation. If we have been trained to focus on patients, we may have neglected the position of friends, family, etc.

It may be painful to reflect

The very notion of 'developing counselling skills' requires us to accept that there is room for improvement in our care. Insightful reflective practice will often require us to think about situations in which we have not helped patients as much as we could have done (Hargreaves 1997). Raising the stakes further, many palliative care situations involve painful symptoms and/or fundamental existential themes and cannot be revisited. Sometimes, reflection will make us realize that we made things worse.

Reflection needs time and practice

Self-reflection and a critical awareness of our own work have to be developed over time. Like any other skill, we are likely to be slower and more self-conscious in the early stages of practising this ability. It follows that counselling skills will be harder to develop in an environment which prizes visible activity and 'doing things' than in an environment which accepts that work may include time to stop and think, or time to discuss experiences with others. If this is not available, staff will find it hard to develop sufficient fluency with self-reflection to make use of this in encounters with patients, rather than in hindsight alone.

Ways to support reflective practice

Use a set of cue questions to structure reflection

Many people find it helpful to build a list of key questions to 'cue' reflection about different aspects of a clinical encounter. At first it may be useful to use a written series of prompts, but in time the HCP will internalize many of these cues and silently begin to ask themselves these questions while talking with patients. Some teams find a short list of cue questions a useful way to structure peer group debriefing, or to develop a more explicitly psychosocial emphasis in handovers. Christopher Johns (1995: 216) suggests questions such as:

'Who is this person?'
'How has this event affected their usual life-patterns and roles?'
'How does this person make me feel?'
'How do they view the future for themselves and others?'

Multidisciplinary reflection

We suggested that one of the blocks to reflective practice are the selective lenses through which we recall events when trying to reflect, and that our professional training is likely to constitute one of these filters. An occupational therapist will tend to notice and understand things differently from a counsellor, who will in turn hear different things in a conversation than will a nurse. We can make positive use of such diversity, and minimize our own blind-spots, by reflecting on clinical situations in multidisciplinary meetings. This may be as a regular part of a palliative care team approach, and/or in response to particularly challenging cases.

Experiential training

We have already suggested that reflection on our clinical practice with patients is a rich resource, but this can be supplemented with other forms of experiential work involving colleagues rather than patients. For example, role-playing clinical situations can provide a forum in which to practise skills, give and receive feedback, and attempt empathic identification with patients through taking on their role. Where money can be found, hiring actors to play patients can give an additional edge to role play, and audio-visual recordings can be made of role-play to aid subsequent review and reflection.

Many people find the very idea of role-play and recordings anxiety-provoking because, quite rightly, they feel 'exposed' to the gaze of others. This is natural, since it signals that experiential work demands a deeper involvement of the whole self beyond simply intellect and memory. This directly parallels the need for good palliative care to follow from engagement between real, whole people, rather then the technical treatment of a sick patient by a healthy professional. There is clearly a need for participants in such workshops to be respectful and supportive towards one another – in itself, another opportunity to practise counselling skills in a very real, emotionally charged context. But if we are not ready to take a small risk in our own training work, how can we ask so much more of patients?

Clinical supervision

Many healthcare professions now recognize a place for clinical supervision in professional development and support, although the manner and degree to which supervision is implemented vary enormously, and there is some disagreement within the field about its functions. Broadly speaking, clinical supervision is a continuing relationship between two or more professionals, in which the designated supervisor aims to help the supervisee(s) to reflect on their work and clinical skills. In some circumstances peers will provide supervision to each other, taking it in turns to be the supervisor/supervisee. In other settings, the supervisor will be a professional who is seen to have more clinical experience and psychosocial expertise and/or specialist supervisory skills. In varying combinations, supervision aims to provide support, to foster learning, and to support the monitoring and maintenance of ethical and professional standards (supportive/restorative, formative and normative roles: Bond and Holland 1998; Hawkins and Shohet 1989).

Clinical supervision can provide a forum in which supervisees can practise their empathic identification with clients and their hypothesizing skills, may develop their capacity to reflect on their own contributions to therapeutic (and counter-therapeutic) processes, and may also provide opportunities to learn and practise new technical skills. A skilled clinical supervisor can enhance the reflective process by encouraging a systematic approach to reflection, supporting the use of intuition and artistry, and providing appropriate challenges or questions concerning apparent 'gaps' or biases in a supervisee's recall of practice.

A programme of personal reading and study

Reading may help us gain a greater empathic understanding of other people's lives which are very different from our own, and also provide us with some conceptual tools to help us develop hypotheses about situations. We have two particular suggestions in developing a reading programme:

- As you read, make an active attempt to link the text with two real patients that you have known, and allow yourself a few moments each time you finish a section to consider how your understanding of those clients and your work with them has been changed by what you have read. You may want to ask yourself what those patients might have said if they had read the same text. Thinking of more than one client may help remind you that any given theoretical concept will vary in its application to different individuals, and help us remain wary of 'one size fits all' conceptualization.
- Read widely. In particular, make a point of reading non-professional accounts of illness and caring, whether these be biographical accounts by patients (Moore 1996), or literary/poetic attempts to explore the human condition and its frailty (Lewis 1966). If we confine ourselves to studying professional texts, we are more likely to approach palliative care issues from a professional-centred viewpoint rather than one which puts us alongside patients (Mooney 1992). This is not in opposition to the modern emphasis on 'evidence-based healthcare'. Instead, we wish to assert the value of patients' illness narratives as an important form of evidence that must be understood in their own terms (Kleinman 1988).

Counselling skills courses

As with any other aspect of professional practice, counselling skills can also be developed through participation in formal courses. These will require a substantial investment of time, and may be costly, so HCPs need to consider carefully how well these fit with their current commitments, and the willingness of their employer to offer study leave and/or funding. It is beyond the scope of this book to review the full range of counselling skills courses available in Britain, but the following points may be useful when trying to select the most appropriate course.

- Will the course offer opportunities to practise and apply skills through experiential work, in addition to any theoretical or didactic teaching? If not, ask yourself carefully whether course attendance will help you any more than a personal programme of study.
- Is the counselling skills course designed specifically for HCPs? If not, will there be other HCPs participating in the course with whom you can share ideas, and who will help to raise issues and examples relevant to your area of practice? If the answer to both these questions is no, there is a risk that you may feel somewhat isolated on the course, and you may have to work extra hard to make connections between the material discussed by others and your own clinical practice. Balanced against this, you might relish the prospect of diversity and fresh thinking from working with people outside your own organization.
- Who will be teaching on the course, and what is their professional background? It is probable that tutors who have a clinical role in a related area of health care will offer a more illuminating experience than tutors whose experience of counselling skills is entirely academic, or relates to professional practice in very different fields (e.g. youth offending and probation).
- Is your aim to develop basic counselling skills applicable to most areas of your practice, or are you relatively confident about this foundation but aiming to extend these skills into less familiar or more challenging areas of palliative care? If the latter, you may feel frustrated on a generic counselling skills course. A number of hospices run education programmes examining specialist aspects of care, such as psychosocial support for children, or supporting the sexual needs of palliative care patients.
- Are you aiming to become a counsellor, or to develop counselling skills to use in your current profession? Courses which aim to provide a qualifying training as a counsellor or psychotherapist are likely to be relatively lengthy and expensive, might not offer a clear focus on healthcare issues, and are subject to complex (and frequently changing) accreditation requirements with national organizations such as the British Association for Counselling, or the United Kingdom Council for Psychotherapy. Given the complex training pathways and

the considerable expense which may be involved, you should seek further advice from these bodies and through consulting texts such as *The Trainee Handbook: A Guide for Counselling and Psychotherapy Trainees* (Robert Bor and Mary Watts, eds, 1999) before making a commitment.

Main learning points

- Listening carefully to feedback from patients and carers is vital in assessing and developing your use of counselling skills.
- Developing and maintaining counselling skills is not simply an individual responsibility, but must be supported through the organizational culture and structures.
- Critical but compassionate reflection on our own clinical practice is one of the most important ways to develop counselling skills.
- Clinical supervision, and/or opportunities for team discussion such as debriefing and multidisciplinary meetings, are valuable ways to support individual attempts at reflective practice.
- There are many different courses on counselling skills. Aim for courses which offer experiential work and some focus on content issues common in palliative care.
- Generic counselling trainings may not be as useful to palliative care workers as specialist counselling skills courses facilitated by HCPs. Consider carefully how you see your future career developing.

Chapter 12

Concluding remarks

Palliative care is an important and expanding area of healthcare in the UK. Although it has historically been closely associated with cancer treatment, there are many patients affected by other serious, progressive and incurable diseases who may also benefit from the palliative emphasis on patients' subjective experience and quality of life.

The rapid development of medical genetics also means that many more people will be living with the knowledge that they carry genetic predispositions to develop serious illnesses, and perhaps that their relatives might also be affected. As medical technology proliferates, so too do the psychological issues involved.

We doubt that increased professional specialization offers a sufficient way forward to meet the emotional and psychological needs of patients and families living with serious illness. We firmly believe that there is a place for specialist counselling. However, each and every encounter with another human being in the healthcare system is potentially helpful or harmful for those affected by illness. Our identities are constructed through our relationships with other people. If these people come to view us simply as symptoms or problems, then both we and they are diminished.

The question is not *whether* we as HCPs need to use counselling and interpersonal skills – this is unavoidable. The issue is whether we use those skills well or badly. It follows that all healthcare workers in palliative care need support to develop and use good counselling skills. In turn, service managers must recognize and support these aspects of caring.

In this book we have chosen to emphasize skills which relate to the HCP's *understandings* of interpersonal encounters, and how these interpretations may guide the supportive roles they adopt towards the person in distress. We hope that this approach offers a useful complement to some other texts which emphasize a more technical, 'micro-skills' approach to counselling skills. We believe that both approaches are important. A capacity for self-reflection and analysis underpins the sensitive selection of responses, while an empathic understanding of a client's situation is of very limited value unless this can be communicated to the client and used to explore further support needs.

We are eager to demystify the term 'counselling skills'. We hope that many of the suggestions and comments in this book will have struck the reader as good 'common sense' and an expression of caring, warm humanity. However, this view contains a trap for the unwary. If we are too ready to rely on our common sense alone, we may fail to recognize differences between ourselves and our clients.

It is possible that this risk may be more marked for experienced palliative care professionals than newly qualified staff. If we believe we are experienced and good at our job through many previous patient contacts, complacency and professional self-confidence may lead us to offer support and services based on our prior experience with those other patients, rather than on an individualized response matched closely to the patient sitting with us here and now.

Good counselling skills may help us hear and learn from patients' feedback more fully, improving evidence-based healthcare by making it less professional-led. This may help each of us develop a better understanding of our own personal 'theory-practice' gap. When we *think* we know what we should do, how can we ensure that this is based on the particular patient's needs rather than professional tradition and routine? Furthermore, how can we account for those occasions when we do understand what the patient needs, and yet we still fail to act on this?

Our intention in this book has been to suggest that good counselling skills are founded on the intentional use of therapeutic relationships. This use must be guided by empathic and contextual insight into the patient's psychological and emotional experience, and linked with a capacity for self-reflection on the part of the HCP. We contend that these are more fundamental considerations than becoming 'word perfect' with particular sequences of questioning or responding, although some forms of wording will communicate more clearly than others.

We have suggested that the development of self-awareness, a capacity for self-reflection, is one of the most important counselling skills. Reflection helps the carer hypothesize about the multiple meanings of what is said and unsaid. It raises our awareness of care issues not only for the patient and their family, but also about our own care needs. Self-reflection is a prerequisite for monitoring our own well-being in a demanding job. In order to care for others we must care for ourselves.

Appendix **A**

Using family genograms

We have emphasized throughout this book that healthcare professionals (HCPs) must work with patients as whole people rather than as problems. To do this, we must work with the family and significant others within the patient's social network, rather than supporting individuals as though they were isolated from a social context.

There are many advantages in developing our understanding of the patient's family context:

- The patient's illness may place those close to them under significant stress. We must assess the support needs of the patient's family and close friends.
- Such assessment helps us understand what care might be provided by family members, without imposing an intolerable or destructive level of carer burden.
- Understanding current and recent events and relationships in the family may help us develop a richer appreciation of the psychological and emotional significance of the patient's illness and symptoms.
- Mapping historical patterns of illness experiences within a family may help us develop hypotheses about the beliefs and coping strategies that the patient and their relatives use to deal with illness (Seaburn *et al.* 1992).

• Demonstrating an interest in the patient's family can be a powerful way to connect with and value the patient, affirming other aspects of their life besides disease.

Experiences of loss are related to the family life-cycle

In trying to understand the losses that an individual and their family may be facing in dealing with serious illness or bereavement, it can be helpful to remember that the meaning of any loss varies in relation to the stage of development that the individual/family is at; the stage of the 'family life cycle' (Carter and McGoldrick 1999). Caring for a partner with a terminal illness may feel very different if the carer also has to care for an elderly dementing parent, than if the carer's parents are relatively young and fit and able to help out.

Families often seem to find it harder to cope with loss through death or illness at times when other changes in family structure have just happened or are about to happen. For example, if cancer strikes a parent when teenage children may be on the point of leaving home, or at a point when marital tensions may have been leading towards a separation, or when someone else in the family has also recently become ill. Sometimes additions to the family (e.g. through marriage, births or adoptions) can seem just as problematic to manage alongside serious illness.

It is as though families need to invest a certain amount of energy and planning into negotiating these 'change points' when the family structure may be altering. Serious illness can take up so much energy and attention that it 'freezes' the planning process for all these other family processes. If the family is unable to find ways to divert some energy and attention to these 'normal' family development issues, as well as to the care of the person who is ill, this can produce considerable tension, frustration, and contribute to a sense that normal family life has been lost.

Helping individuals and families to talk about and plan for some of these 'normal' family issues can sometimes be a powerful way to restore some of the loss that the illness has threatened. This applies particularly if other conversations with professionals are focusing exclusively on the illness itself and on care arrangements, rather than on the rest of the patient's and family's life together.

Using genograms focuses attention on family systems issues

Some palliative care units have begun to use genograms as a way to support systematic reflection on the patient in their family context. A genogram is a kind of 'family tree' which records information about family structure, relationships and significant dates and events in a diagrammatic form (McGoldrick and Gerson 1985). Such information can of course be recorded in other forms, but genograms:

- are easier to study as a whole and take in 'at a glance';
- make it easier to spot patterns within families, especially if combined with a 'time-line' summarizing significant dates and 'coincidences' between particular kinds of anniversary;
- can be added to and fleshed out more easily as new information emerges, providing a useful working 'team' document; and
- are readily understood during interviews by many patients and relatives as family trees, providing a powerful stimulus to discussion and the exploration of illness experiences.

Constructing a genogram with a patient and/or relative

- Avoid jargon. Describe the genogram as a family tree.
- Explain to the patient why you are interested in their family and how this might be helpful.
- Start simply. Begin with factual questions about dates, names and places (e.g. who was born when and where, who died when and of what?). Remember to ask about and record information about family members who have died, rather than simply list relatives still living.

Drawing a genogram with a patient needs sensitivity like any other caring interaction. Attend to the patient's feelings and

People

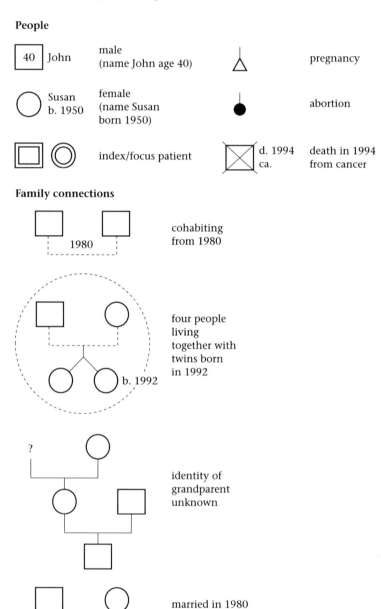

40 John	male (name John age 40)	pregnancy
Susan b. 1950	female (name Susan born 1950)	abortion
□ ◎	index/focus patient	d. 1994 ca. — death in 1994 from cancer

Family connections

cohabiting from 1980

four people living together with twins born in 1992

identity of grandparent unknown

married in 1980

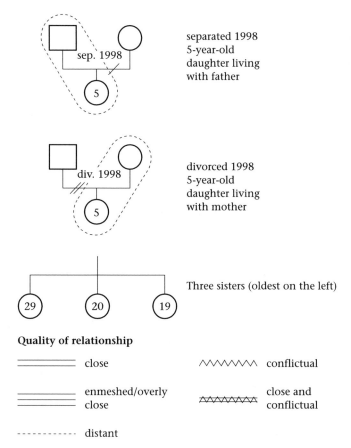

separated 1998
5-year-old
daughter living
with father

divorced 1998
5-year-old
daughter living
with mother

Three sisters (oldest on the left)

Quality of relationship

close   conflictual

enmeshed/overly
close   close and
                               conflictual

distant

Figure 3 Genogram symbols

responses. Let this guide the pace of the interview. It may be appropriate to construct or add to the genogram over several conversations, rather than treat it as a 'timed test' that has to be finished in one session.

The aim is not to get as much information as possible. The purpose is to understand and relate to the patient and their family better. It is valuable to notice which aspects the patient finds it *hard* to discuss, without pushing the patient to reveal details they would prefer to keep private.

As the genogram develops, add questions about the

meaning of events and how relationships in the family have changed over time or been affected by illness events.

- Invite the patient to explain in their own words, like telling a story. Avoid closed questions seeking only short answers.
- Ask patients with partners about *both* families.
- Seek information about at least three generations. This helps to tap into enduring patterns and beliefs in families about coping with illness.
- Thank the patient for helping the team.

Some questions to consider when reviewing genograms

1 What kind of illnesses has this family had to deal with in the past? What coping strategies did they use, and how well did these work?
2 Might the family need support to recognize some of the different demands of the current illness, or support to remember and apply successful strategies used with similar illnesses?
3 What previous dealings have family members had with health-care professionals? How might this influence their expectations of current HCPs?
4 Are there other changes (e.g. divorces, redundancies, pregnancy) and/or health events in the family at present which may add to the patient's concerns, or mean that coping resources in the family may be thinly stretched?
5 Who might be most isolated or vulnerable following bereavement? How has the family dealt with previous bereavements?
6 When considering any palliative care situation involving a couple, how might their *different* family histories affect their attitudes to illness and their capacity to agree their approach to living with illness? (Has the couple ever had to do this before?)
7 How might the cultural and religious background of the family affect the care that the HCPs need to provide?
8 Are there other people who are very important to the patient who are not included in the genogram? (Note that attention to such issues is important in ensuring that gay and lesbian

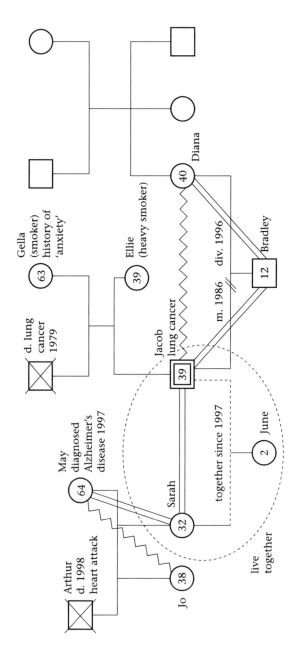

Figure 4 An example of a genogram

relationships, and less 'conventional' relationships are adequately recognized and valued. There is a danger in asking about 'family' relationships that this can be interpreted too narrowly by patient, HCP or both.)

Reviewing this genogram (Figure 4) makes us think, for example, about:

- the possible impact of repeated losses and multiple carer burdens on Sarah;
- the sort of health advice that should be offered to Ellie and Gella;
- how Jacob's expectations of cancer are shaped by his father's experience of illness;
- how contacts between Bradley and Jacob can be negotiated sensitively.

Appendix **B**

Contacts and resources

Association of Palliative Medicine (APM)

The APM is a member of the European Association of Palliative Care and is an association of doctors who work in hospices and specialist palliative care units. The Association exists to promote the advancement and development of palliative medicine for the terminally ill through an information newsletter and the development of education and training materials, study days and dissemination of information through a database of doctors working within the speciality to assist with staffing and training requirements.

Association of Palliative Medicine
11 Westwood Road
Southampton
Hampshire SO1 1DL
Phone: (023) 8067 2888
Email: apmsecretariat@claranet.co.uk

The British Association for Counselling (BAC)

The Association aims to promote the understanding and aware-ness of counselling and represents counselling at national and international levels. The Association also responds to requests for information and advice on matters related to counselling and provides opportunities for the continual professional development of counsellors and support for those using counselling skills.

The British Association for Counselling
1 Regent Place
Rugby
Warwickshire CV21 2PJ
Phone: (01788) 550899
Fax: (01788) 562189
Email: bac@bac.co.uk

CancerBACUP

CancerBACUP aims to help people live with cancer by providing information and emotional support to patients, their families and health professionals. It is one of the foremost providers of cancer information in the UK.

CancerBACUP
3 Bath Place
Rivington Street
London EC2A 3DR
Phone: (020) 7613 2121
Fax: (020) 7696 9002
Email: info@cancerbacup.org

Help the Hospices

Help the Hospices is an umbrella organization set up to provide financial support to ensure that all hospices continue to provide the best possible palliative care. This includes funding for training courses to charitable and NHS palliative care units and nursing homes, and covers a range of specialist courses for doctors and nurses, training for clergy, counsellors and many other professions within the palliative care team. This charitable organization raises money to support hospices by providing equipment for patient care, pump priming funds for key posts and research into care and treatment.

Help the Hospices
34–44 Britannia Street
London WC1X 9JG
Phone: (020) 7278 5668
Fax: (020) 7278 1021
Email: info@helpthehospices.org.uk

The Hospice Information Service at St Christopher's

The Hospice Information Service is part of a joint development between St Christopher's Hospice and King's College London, and provides a worldwide link to encourage sharing of information and experience among those involved in palliative care. The Service produces a *Hospice Directory*, which outlines facts and figures of palliative care provision in the UK. It also produces a quarterly newsletter, which includes up-to-date information, UK and international news, research, video and book reviews. The publication *Choices* is a comprehensive source of information on training opportunities in palliative care and bereavement.

Hospice Information Service
St Christopher's Hospice
51–59 Lawrie Park Road
London SE26 6DZ
Phone: (020) 8778 9252
Fax: (020) 8776 9345
Email: his@stchris.ftech.co.uk

The Lesbian and Gay Bereavement Project

The Lesbian and Gay Bereavement Project is a charitable organization which provides support and help for lesbians and gay men through the bereavement of their partner and any person who is suffering bereavement following the death of a lesbian or gay man. The Lesbian and Gay Bereavement Project offers individuals one-to-one counselling sessions with their trained counsellors. The Project also offers education about same gender loss to professionals working with the bereaved and dying.

The Lesbian and Gay Bereavement Project
Vaughan M. Williams Centre
Colindale Hospital
Colindale Avenue
London NW9 5HG
Phone: (020) 8200 0511
Email: lgbp@aol.com

The Motor Neurone Disease Association

The Motor Neurone Disease (MND) Association is funded entirely from voluntary donations and was formed to bring together all those people concerned with MND, including those living with the disease, their carers, and health and social care professionals. The Association aims to secure care and support for people affected by MND and to raise awareness and understanding of the disease in addition to promoting research within the field.

MND Association UK
PO Box 246
Northampton NN1 2PR
Phone: (01604) 250505
Fax: (01604) 624726

The National Council for Hospice and Specialist Palliative Care Services (NCHSPCS)

The National Council's role is to represent the views and interests of hospice organizations and palliative care services and to provide a forum to share knowledge, information and experience. The NCHSPCS also publishes regular information about the work of the Council and develops professional standards, audit and policies as a means through which care provision is coordinated and professional education and research encouraged.

The National Council for Hospice and Specialist Palliative Care
Services
34–44 Britannia Street
London WC1X 9JG
Phone: (020) 7520 8299
Email: enquiries@hospice-spc-council.org.uk

The National HIV Nurses' Association (NHIVNA)

The NHIVNA provides a national network for all nurses working in the care of people with HIV throughout the UK and aims to provide an academic and educational forum for the dissemination of original nursing research in the field of HIV/AIDS. In addition to this the Association also aims to address the communication and support needs of nurses working in this area, to assist in the promotion of good practice in the care of people with HIV.

National HIV Nurses' Association
The Foundation of Nursing Studies
32 Buckingham Palace Road
London SW1W 0RE
Phone: (020) 7233 5750
Fax: (020) 7233 5759
Email: admin@fons.org

Nurseline and the Royal College of Nursing (RCN) Counselling and Advisory Service

Nurseline is an advisory service for all nurses and midwives, including students and those retired from the profession, provided by the RCN with the Lisa Sainsbury Foundation. Callers are referred to the most appropriate source of help and information; the service has particular expertise in housing, grant aid, finance and career advice. The RCN Counselling and Advisory Service offers free, professional and confidential counselling to RCN members on personal or work-related issues.

Nurseline and the Royal College of Nursing Counselling and
  Advisory Service
8–10 Crown Hill
Croydon CR0 1RZ
Phone: (020) 8681 4030
Email: nursingstandard@compuserve.com

*The Association to Aid the Sexual and Personal
Relationships of People with a Disability (SPOD)*

The Association to Aid the Sexual and Personal Relationships of
  People with a Disability (SPOD)
286 Camden Road
London N7 0BJ
Phone: (020) 7607 8851

The Tavistock Institute

The Tavistock Institute is an independent not-for-profit organization, which seeks to combine research in the social sciences with professional practice. The Institute is entirely self-financing, with no subsidies from the government or other sources. Its action research orientation places it between, but not in, the worlds of academia and consultancy; and its range of disciplines include anthropology, economics, organizational behaviour, political science, psychoanalysis, psychology and sociology.

The Tavistock Institute
30 Tabernacle Street
London EC2A 4DD
Phone: (020) 7417 0407
Fax: (020) 7417 0566
Email: central.admin@tavinstitute.org

Training material contacts

Concord Video and Film Council
201 Felixstowe Road
Ipswich
Suffolk IP3 9BJ
Phone: (01473) 726012

DMP Productions and CEC
Hebron Hall
Cross Common Road
Dinas Powys
South Wales
CF64 4YB
Phone/Fax: (01222) 514831

FEPI/Family Experiences Productions, Inc.
PO Box 5879
Austin, TX 78763-5879
Phone: 00 1 512 494 0338
Fax: 00 1 512 494 0340
Email: fepirag@aol.com

Linkward Productions Limited
Post 63
Shepperton Studio Centre
Squires
Shepperton
Middlesex TW17 0QD

Pavilion Publishing (Brighton) Limited
8 St George's Place
Brighton
East Sussex BN1 4GB
Phone: (01273) 623222
Fax: (01273) 625526
Email: pavpub@pavilion.co.uk

TCA Consulting
Southpoint
8 Paston Place
Brighton
East Sussex BN2 1HA
Phone: (01273) 693622
Fax: (01273) 670487

References

Altschuler, J. (1997) *Working with Chronic Illness*. Basingstoke: Macmillan.

Anon. (1991) *Mud and Stars*. Report of a Working Party on the Impact of Hospice Experience on the Church's Ministry of Healing. Oxford: Sobell Publications.

Barry, P. D. (1996) *Psychosocial Nursing: Care of Physically Ill Patients and Their Families*. Philadelphia, PA: Lippincott.

Benner, P. and Wrubel, J. (1989) *The Primacy of Caring: Stress and Coping in Health and Illness*. Menlo Park, CA: Addison-Wesley.

Biswas, B. (1993) The medicalization of dying: a nurse's view, in D. Clark (ed.) *The Future of Palliative Care*. Buckingham: Open University Press.

Bond, M. and Holland, S. (1998) *Skills of Clinical Supervision for Nurses*. Buckingham: Open University Press.

Bor, R. and Watts, M. (eds) (1999) *The Trainee Handbook: A Guide for Counselling and Psychotherapy Trainees*. London: Sage.

Bor, R., Miller, R., Latz, M. and Salt, H. (1998) *Counselling in Health Care Settings*. London and New York: Cassell.

Bright, R. (1998) *Grief and Powerlessness: Helping People Regain Control of Their Life*. London: Jessica Kingsley.

Burnham, J. (1986) *Family Therapy: First Steps towards a Systemic Approach*. London and New York: Routledge.

Burton, M. and Watson. M. (1998) *Counselling People with Cancer*. London: Wiley.

Carter, B. and McGoldrick, M. (eds) (1999) *The Extended Family Life-Cycle*, 3rd edn. New York: Gardiner Press.

Cecchin, G. (1987) Hypothesising, circularity and neutrality revisited: an invitation to curiosity, *Family Process*, 26: 405–13.

Corby, B. (1993) *Child Abuse: Towards a Knowledge Base*. Buckingham: Open University Press.

das Gupta, P. (1994) Images of childhood and theories of development, in J. Oates (ed.) *The Foundations of Child Development*. Buckingham: Open University Press.

Davy, J. (1999) A biopsychosocial approach to counselling in primary care, in R. Bor and D. McCann (eds) *The Practice of Counselling in Primary Care*. London: Sage.

de Shazer, S. (1984) The death of resistance, *Family Process*, 23: 11–17.

Dickenson, D. and Johnson, M. (1993) *Death, Dying and Bereavement*. London: Sage.

Ellis, S. (1997) Research and development: patient and professional centred care in the hospice, *International Journal of Palliative Nursing*, 3(4): 197–202.

Faulkner, A. and Maguire, P. (1994) *Talking to Cancer Patients and Their Relatives*. Oxford: Oxford Medical Publications.

Fredman, G. (1997) *Death Talk: Conversations with Children and Families*. London: Karnac.

George, E., Iveson, C. and Ratner, H. (1990) *Problem to Solution: Brief Therapy with Individuals and Families*. London: BT Press.

Hargreaves, J. (1997) Using patients: exploring the ethical dimension of reflective practice in nurse education, *Journal of Advanced Nursing*, 25(2): 223–8.

Hawkins, P. and Shohet, R. (1989) *Supervision in the Helping Professions*. Milton Keynes: Open University Press.

Herbert, M. (1996) *Supporting Bereaved and Dying Children and Their Parents*. Leicester: BPS Books.

Imber-Black, E., Roberts, J. and Whiting. R. (eds) (1988) *Rituals in Families and Family Therapy*. New York: Norton.

Johns, C. (1995) Framing learning through reflection within Carper's fundamental ways of knowing in nursing, *Journal of Advanced Nursing*, 22(2): 226–34.

Johns, C. (1998) Opening the doors of perception, in C. Johns and D. Freshwater (eds) *Transforming Nursing through Reflective Practice*. Oxford: Blackwell.

Jones, E. (1993) *Family Systems Therapy: Developments in the Milan-Systemic Therapies*. Chichester: Wiley.

Judd, D. (1989) *Give Sorrow Words: Working with a Dying Child*. London: Free Association Books.

Kearney, A. (1996) *Mortally Wounded: Stories of Soul Pain, Death and Healing*. Dublin: Marino.

Kleinman, A. (1988) *The Illness Narratives: Suffering, Healing and the Human Condition*. New York: Basic Books.

Lawler, J. (1991) *Behind the Screens: Nursing, Somology and the Problem of the Body*. Singapore: Churchill Livingstone.

Lazarus, R. S. and Folkman, S. (1984) *Stress, Appraisal, and Coping*. New York: Springer Publications.

Lederberg, M. (1990) Psychological problems of staff and their management, in J. Holland and J. Rowland (eds) *Handbook of Psychooncology*. Oxford: Oxford Medical Press.

Lemma, A. (1997) *An Introduction to Psychopathology*. Chichester: Wiley.

Lewis, C. S. (1966) *A Grief Observed*. London: Faber.

MacElveen-Hoehn, P. (1985) Sexual assessment and counselling, *Seminars in Oncology Nursing*, 1(1): 69–75.

Maslach, C. (1981) *Burnout: The Cost of Caring*. Englewood Cliffs, NJ: Prentice Hall.

McGoldrick, M. and Gerson, R. (1985) *Genograms in Family Assessment*. New York: Basic Books.

Menzies Lyth, I. (1988) [1957] The functioning of social systems as a defence against anxiety, in I. Menzies Lyth, *Containing Anxiety in Institutions: Selected Essays*. London: Free Association Books.

Miller, S. D., Duncan, B. L. and Hubble, M. A. (1997) *Escape from Babel: Toward a Unifying Language for Psychotherapy Practice*. London: Norton.

Mooney, B. (1992) *Perspectives for Living: Conversations on Bereavement and Love*. London: John Murray.

Moore, O. (1996) *Person With AIDS: Looking Aids in the Face*. London: Picador.

NCHSPCS (1993) *Key Ethical Issues in Palliative Care: Evidence to the House of Lords Select Committee on Medical Ethics*. London: National Council for Hospice and Specialist Palliative Care Services.

NCHSPCS (1995) *Specialist Palliative Care: A Statement of Definitions*. London: National Council for Hospice and Specialist Palliative Care Services.

NCHSPCS (1997) *Voluntary Euthanasia: The Council's View*. London: National Council for Hospice and Specialist Palliative Care Services.

Nordman, T., Kasen, A. and Eriksson, K. (1998) Reflective practice: a way to the patient's world and Caring, the core of nursing, in C. Johns and D. Freshwater (eds) *Transforming Nursing through Reflective Practice*. Oxford: Blackwell Science.

Nuland, S. B. (1993) *How We Die*. London: Chatto and Windus.

O'Berle, K. and Davies, B. (1990) Dimensions of the supportive role of the nurse in palliative care, *Oncology Nursing Forum*, 17: 87–94.

O'Berle, K. and Davies, B. (1992) Support and caring: exploring the concepts, *Oncology Nursing Forum*, 19(5): 763–7.

Obholzer, A. and Roberts, V. (1994) *The Unconscious at Work: Individual and Organisational Stress in the Human Services*. London: Routledge.

van Ooijen, E. (1996) Learning to approach patients' sexuality as part of holistic care, *Nursing Times*, 92(36): 4 September.

Parkes, C. M. and Hinde, J. (1982) *The Place of Attachment in Human Behaviour*. London: Tavistock Publications.

Parkes, C. M., Relf, M. and Couldrick, A. (1996) *Counselling in Terminal Care and Bereavement*. Leicester: BPS.

Price, B. (1995) Assessing altered body image, *Journal of Psychiatric and Mental Health Nursing*, 2: 169–75.

Riches, G. and Dawson, P. (2000) *An Intimate Loneliness: Supporting Bereaved Parents and Siblings*. Buckingham: Open University Press.

Rogers, C. R. (1957) The necessary and sufficient conditions of therapeutic personality change, *Journal of Consulting Psychology*, 21: 95–103.

Rolland, J. (1994) *Families, Illness and Disability*. New York: Basic Books.

Russell, G. and Hersov, L. (1983) *Handbook of Psychiatry*, 4: 205–6. Cambridge: Cambridge University Press.

Salter, M. (1997) *Altered Body Image: The Nurse's Role*. London: Ballière Tindall.

Seaburn, D., Lorenz, A. and Kaplan, D. (1992) The transgenerational development of chronic illness meanings, *Family Systems Medicine*, 10: 385–95.

Speck, P. (1996) Unconscious communication, *Palliative Medicine*, 10: 273–4.

Stedeford, A. (1994) *Facing Death: Patients, Families and Professionals*. Oxford: Sobell Publications.

Stroebe, M. S., Stroebe, W. and Hanson, R. O. (1992) *Handbook of Bereavement: Theory, Research and Intervention*. Cambridge: Cambridge University Press.

Stroebe, W. and Stroebe, M. S. (1995) *Social Psychology and Health*. Buckingham: Open University Press.

Tebbitt, P. (1999) *Palliative Care 2000: Commissioning through Partnership*. Northamptonshire: National Council for Hospice and Specialist Palliative Care Services.

Tschudin, V. (1987) *Counselling Skills for Nurses*, 2nd edn. London: Ballière Tindall.

Walter, T. (2000) *On Bereavement: The Culture of Grief*. Buckingham: Open University Press.

White, M. (1989) The Externalising of the Problem, *Dulwich Centre Newsletter*, Special edn.

Woodruff, R. (1997) *Cancer Pain*. Victoria: Asperula.

Woolfe, R. and Dryden, W. (1996) *Handbook of Counselling Psychology*. London: Sage.

Wright, L., Watson, W. and Bell, J. (1996) *Beliefs: The Heart of Healing in Families and Illness*. New York: Basic Books.

Yalom, I. D. (1989) *Love's Executioner and Other Tales of Psychotherapy*. London: Penguin.

Index

alliances, 21
ambiguity, 3, 91, 92
anger, 77–8, 83–98, 129–31
assessment, 24, 30
avoidance, 7–8, 63, 101, 141

bereavement, 123–33
brevity, 117, 141
British Association for
    Counselling (BAC), 156

child protection, 104–5
children, 99–110
choice, 11, 34–5, 48, 58, 102,
    120–1
closure, 61, 74
compassion, 85–6
complacency, 118, 159
confidentiality, 104–5, 110
connecting, 14, 18–19, 25–6, 27,
    57–8, 100–1, 119–20
containing, 21–2, 30, 58
context, 13, 36–7, 161–2
coping, 46–7
coping strategies, 38–40, 48
counselling skills
  common factors, 13–14
  definition, 12–15

and other forms of support, 35
courses in counselling skills,
    155–7
culture, 150–1
curiosity, 34, 65–6, 73

death, 12, 111–22, 125–8, 131–2,
    139–40
dilemmas, 102–3
dimensions of relationship,
    14–15, 51
  see also connecting, 'doing for',
    empowering, integrity,
    meaning-finding, valuing
disclosure, 54, 56–8, 68, 72–3,
    105
disease, and illness, 42, 79–80
distress, 23–6
'doing for', 14, 51, 91–3

empathy, 33–7, 47, 57, 77, 146
empowering, 14, 31–48, 91–2,
    119
escalation, 84–7, 95–7
euthanasia, 75–8, 81–2
existential dilemmas, 11–12
  see also choice, death,
    isolation, meaninglessless

expert status, 60
externalizing, 87

faith, 64–7
family life-cycle, 43, 162–3
fatigue, 107–8
fear, 18–20, 47–8, 54–8, 72–3,
    78–9, 120–1
feelings, 22, 33, 54–8, 77–8, 96–7
'fight or flight', 85, 95, 98

genograms, 161–8
goals, of client, 13
gratitude, 130–1, 142–4, 147
guilt, 110

holistic approach, 27, 79–80, 123,
    125
hope, 13
hospice movement, history, 3–6
hypothesizing, 34, 48, 90–1,
    107–8, 149

integrity, 14–15, 52, 76, 95–7
isolation, 11

listening, 24–5, 30, 54–6, 73, 149
loss, 49–68, 162–3

meaning-finding, 14, 103, 113–14
meaninglessness, 11
multidisciplinary team work, 8–9,
    141–2

neutrality, 21, 29, 36–7, 40, 45,
    76–7, 101–2, 110, 129
non-judgemental attitude, 13,
    39–40, 48, 85–6
normalization, 20, 25, 47

pain, 78–81
palliative care
    and curative treatment, 3, 17

definition, 2–3
history, 3–6
patient-centred approach, 50–1,
    57–8, 63, 72, 116
PLISSIT, 60
proactive intervention, 27, 41–2
psychosocial issues, 42–3, 54

questions
    coping, 46–7
    open/closed/leading, 73, 105

reassurance, false, 18–19, 33, 47,
    101, 113–14
referral, 27–9, 44, 57, 60, 104
reflection, 39–40, 85–6, 151–5,
    157, 160
relationship, 12, 13, 14–15, 54,
    100–1, 112–13, 121, 160
resistance, 88
resources, of client, 13, 65–6
risk assessment, 28–9
Royal College of Physicians, 6

Saunders, Cicely, 3, 4
skills
    development, 148–57
    vs. techniques, 13–14, 112–
    13
suicide and self harm, 75, 81–2
supervision, 154
symptoms, 69–82, 161

touch, 25–6, 119–20
transference, 91
trust, 51, 68, 81

United Kingdom Council for
    Psychotherapy (UKCP), 156

validation, 25, 47, 51, 54–8,
    96–7
valuing, 13, 14, 51, 77, 109, 114